POWERFUL
PLANT~BASED
SUPER
FOODS

For Maria

IIIIIIIIIIIIIIIIIIIIIIIIIIIIIIIIIIIIIIII

© 2013 Fair Winds Press
Text © 2013 Lauri Boone
Photography © 2013 Fair Winds Press

First published in the USA in 2013 by
Fair Winds Press, a member of
Quayside Publishing Group
100 Cummings Center
Suite 406-L
Beverly, MA 01915-6101
www.fairwindspress.com

17 16 15 14 13   2 3 4 5

ISBN: 978-1-59233-534-3

Digital edition published in 2013
eISBN: 978-1-61058-749-5

Library of Congress Cataloging-in-Publication Data
Boone, Lauri.
  Powerful plant-based superfoods : the best way to eat for maximum health, energy, and weight loss / Lauri Boone.
     pages cm
  Includes index.
  ISBN 978-1-59233-534-3
  1. Weight loss. 2. Cooking (Natural foods) 3. Cooking (Vegetables) I. Title.
  RM222.2.B632 2013
  641.3'02--dc23
                         2012037438

Cover and Book design by Laura McFadden

Photography by Bill Bettencourt
Food Styling by Lynne Aloia

Shutterstock.com: 4, 5, 7, 8, 9, 11, 12, 16, 18, 20, 22, 24, 26, 28, 30, 32, 34, 36, 38, 40, 42, 44, 46, 47, 49, 50, 52, 54, 56, 58,
60, 62, 64, 66, 68, 69, 71, 74, 76, 78, 80, 81, 84, 88, 89, 92, 93, 95, 96, 98, 100, 102, 108, 110, 114, 117, 118, 119, 122, 124, 126, 128,
130, 132, 136, 138, 140, 144, 147, 148, 150, 152, 154, 156, 157, 162, 166, 168, 170, 172, 174, 175, 177, 178, 180, 182, 184, 185, 188,
190, 192, 194, 196, 198, 201, 202, 204, 205, 207, 208, 214
E3Live: 90, 134
Fotolia: 112
Funky Stock, Paul Williams/Alamy: 142
Sacha Vida: page 164

Printed and bound in China

The information in this book is for educational purposes only. It is not intended to replace the advice of a physician
or medical practitioner. Please see your health care provider before beginning any new health program.

POWERFUL PLANT~BASED SUPER FOODS

The Best Way to Eat for Maximum Health, Energy, and Weight Loss

LAURI BOONE, R.D.

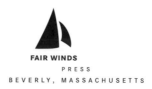

FAIR WINDS
PRESS
BEVERLY, MASSACHUSETTS

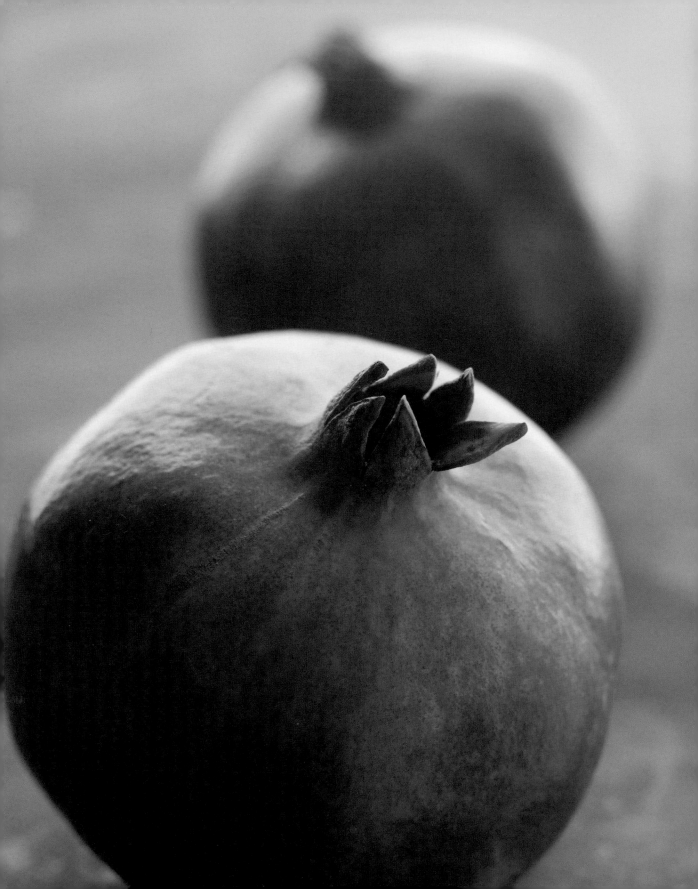

CONTENTS

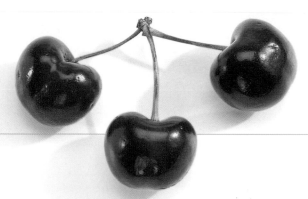

INTRODUCTION

Here is the plain-and-simple truth about your diet: You are what you eat. As often as you hear these words, have you ever stopped to think about the significance of them? Food has the impressive ability to affect—for better or worse—every cell and system in your body, and every time you eat you are making a choice for your mind, body, and spirit. Your food choices can make you feel tired and bloated or light and energized. They can help you stay calm and clear or feel foggy and frazzled. They can help keep your body slim and skin glowing or cause weight gain and breakouts.

What you put in your body has a significant bearing on your overall health and vitality, and the fact that food can influence your health so radically is great news indeed. It means that you can harness the power of food and use it to heal and protect your body both inside and out. And you can start right now—with superfoods.

The Magic of Superfoods

One of the simplest ways to upgrade your diet is by adding superfoods. Superfoods are the most nutrient-dense foods in the world. They are real, whole, unprocessed, plant-based foods that are packed with a wide array of health-promoting compounds, including remarkable levels of vitamins and minerals, inflammation-fighting fats, easy-to-digest proteins, and heart-healthy fiber. The plant-based superfoods in this book are also rich in a variety of phytochemicals (active compounds found only in plant foods) and cell-protecting antioxidants, which help combat the cell-damaging effects of free radicals (see sidebar "Amazing Antioxidants" for more information).

From familiar foods like blueberries and kale to lesser-known ones like açai and maca, these superstars (and the combination of beneficial compounds in them) may help reduce inflammation, slow aging, prevent or treat chronic disease, increase energy, boost mood, reduce stress, cleanse the body by supporting its natural detoxification pathways, and so much more. Superfoods are not magic bullets, but they are pretty magical.

Building a Superfood Diet

Superfoods offer up a pretty impressive list of benefits to mind and body—and the fifty plant-based superfoods in this book include some of the top present and emerging foods for peak health. In fact, you could say these foods are the "cream of the crop." But as I mentioned, superfoods are not magical cure-alls for whatever might be ailing you—at least not when consumed in the context of an overall lousy diet full

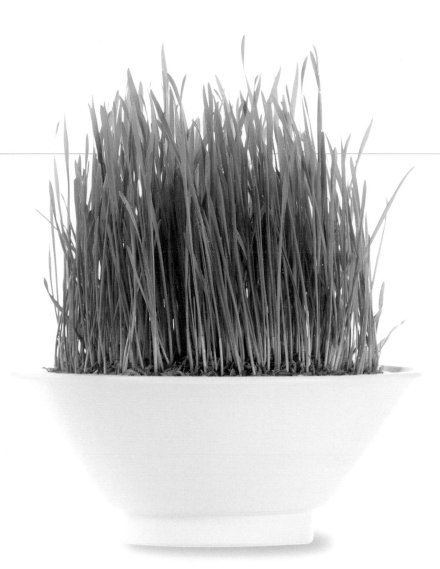

AMAZING ANTIOXIDANTS

Antioxidants are compounds (including vitamins like vitamins C and E; minerals like selenium; and phytochemicals like beta-carotene) that help quench the activities of free radicals, unstable molecules that can damage your body's cells. Free radicals are produced as normal by-products of metabolism and by external factors, such as your lifestyle choices. A poor diet (too much processed food, sugar, caffeine, and alcohol) excessive exercise, poor sleep, emotional stress, and exposure to environmental toxins can all drive the production of free radicals in the body.

And when your body produces more free radicals than it can handle, oxidative stress occurs, setting the stage for diseases like cancer, heart disease, diabetes, and even brain and autoimmune disorders. Just as a car left outside to weather the elements will rust, so will your body when left unprotected. Eating antioxidant-rich superfoods can help combat the cell-damaging effects of free radicals and fight inflammation. And as researchers are still learning, antioxidants also appear to have beneficial non-antioxidant activities (outside of their ability to scavenge free radicals) that may contribute to their potential health benefits.

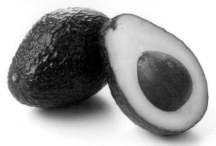

of processed and junk foods. If you want to really make significant changes to your health and well-being, you need to make good choices, consistently and consciously—one meal and snack at a time.

SUPERFOODS ARE FOR EVERYONE

Whether you define your diet as raw, vegan, vegetarian, omnivore, conscious carnivore, or perhaps you don't define your diet at all—this book and the superfoods in it are for you. With practical tips and a mix of simple raw and cooked food recipes, anyone—and I mean anyone—can begin to work with the fifty plant-based superfoods on these pages. In fact, incorporating small amounts of these nutrient-dense foods into your daily diet will give it a huge and healthy upgrade.

Superfood Rules

Before you dive into the magic of superfoods, take a moment to read a few of my superfood rules to help you get the most from your diet and this book.

- **Eat real food.** More than forty-eight thousand foods and food products line the shelves of the average American supermarket. Foods that come in boxes and bags or with lengthy lists of hard-to-decipher ingredients are not real foods and do not offer much nutrition. So start filling your plate with real food, and limit or avoid eating from a can, box, or bag. The recipes in this book will help you get started!

- **Eat more plants.** Everyone benefits from eating more plant foods. Foods that grow on a tree or out of the ground—such as vegetables, fruits, sprouts, legumes (beans, peas, and lentils), nuts, and seeds—should form the foundation of your diet. Experiment freely with the fifty plant-based superfoods in this book!

EWG'S 2012 *SHOPPER'S GUIDE TO PESTICIDES IN PRODUCE*

Dirty Dozen Plus ||||||||||||||||||||||||||||||||||||||||||||||||

1. Apples
2. Celery
3. Sweet bell peppers
4. Peaches
5. Strawberries
6. Nectarines, imported
7. Grapes
8. Spinach
9. Lettuce
10. Cucumbers
11. Blueberries, domestic
12. Potatoes
+Green beans
+ Kale/greens

Clean 15 ||||||||||||||||||||||||||||||||||||||||||||||||

1. Onions
2. Sweet corn
3. Pineapples
4. Avocados
5. Cabbage
6. Sweet peas
7. Asparagus
8. Mangoes
9. Eggplant
10. Kiwi
11. Cantaloupe, domestic
12. Sweet potatoes
13. Grapefruit
14. Watermelon
15. Mushrooms

CHOOSING ORGANIC FRUITS AND VEGETABLES

Don't be deterred from filling up on fruits and vegetables if you can't find or afford organic produce. The Environmental Working Group's (EWG) popular *Shopper's Guide to Pesticides in Produce* will assist you in choosing between organic and conventional. Published annually, this guide includes a list of the Dirty Dozen Plus (the twelve most heavily contaminated fruits and vegetables, plus crops that may not meet the Dirty Dozen criteria but have high contamination levels) and the Clean 15 (the fifteen least-contaminated fruits and vegetables). Many of the superfoods in this book, as well as ingredients in accompanying recipes, are on these lists. You can lower your pesticide intake by choosing conventional for the least contaminated produce, and choosing organic for the most heavily contaminated produce.

- **Buy seasonal and local food.** Choosing local and seasonal food is good for your health and the health of the planet. The average meal travels about 1,500 miles (2,414 kilometers) from farm to plate, and while your food is being shipped across the country or overseas, it loses valuable nutrients and wastes precious resources. So choose local food most often. You can grow your own food, buy from a farmers' market, or join a local CSA (community-supported agriculture)—check out the resources section of this book for more information. And although these pages include some pretty exotic but easy-to-find foods, if you look around, you will find plenty of superfoods growing right in your own backyard.

- **Choose organic.** Buying organic ensures that the food you eat is produced without conventional pesticides, fertilizers made with synthetic ingredients or sewage sludge (that's right, sewage sludge), ionizing radiation, or bioengineering (just say no to genetically modified foods). And if you consume animal products, choosing organic ensures that they have not been treated with antibiotics or growth hormones—both of which can be passed along to you. Remember, you are what you eat—so eat more plants and choose organic when available.

- **Give your diet a superfood boost.** Ready to upgrade your diet? Filling your plate with nutrient-, antioxidant-, and phytochemical-rich superfoods will give your diet a big boost—and that's where the practical tips and recipes in this book come into action. Although there are no hard-and-fast rules for how many servings of superfoods you should be eating—everyone's nutritional needs and preferences are highly unique—I challenge you to incorporate at least one or two of these foods into your diet each and every day for a superfood and super nutrient boost. Your body will thank you.

- **Eat for pleasure.** Finally, food should taste good. Period. Lucky for you, real food does taste good, and once you start filling up on real food—like the superfoods in this book—you will find yourself craving them more. And even better, the recipes in this book require minimal ingredients, equipment, and preparation (aside from some soaking here and there), which makes it easy for you to find pleasure in creating meals and snacks, too (because let's face it, not everyone wants to spend their time searching for hard-to-find ingredients or cooking all day in the kitchen).

Are you ready? Let's get started!

CHOOSE FOOD, NOT SUPPLEMENTS

There are lots of superfood supplements on the market, but I want you to eat real superfoods—not take superfood supplements. The nutrients in food appear to work synergistically to benefit our body, and supplements do not always have the same effect as whole foods. With a few exceptions (such as AFA blue-green algae, spirulina, and chlorella), the superfoods in this book are typically found in their whole food form. And they are super tasty and super simple to add to your everyday diet. So go ahead and toss some açai pulp into your smoothies, crush a little extra garlic into your salads and soups, curl up with a cup of green tea—and make friends with real food. An additional bonus: The money you save on supplements can be spent on organic food!

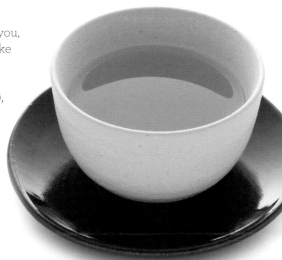

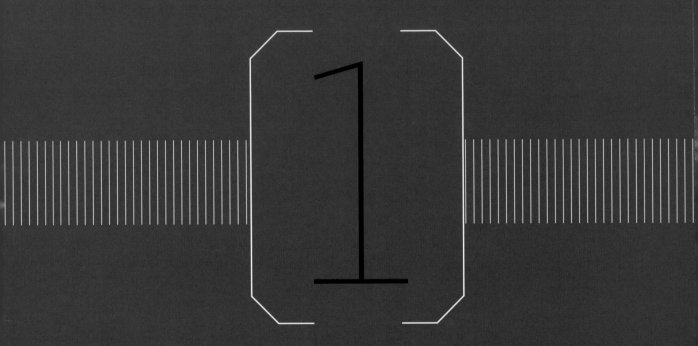

1

SUPER BERRIES

Açai Berry, Blueberry, Camu Camu Berry, Cranberry, Goji Berry, Goldenberry, Maqui Berry, Mulberry, Sea Buckthorn Berry

Berries are the ultimate antiaging superfoods. They top the charts with their high levels of antioxidants and phytochemicals to keep your brain young, skin glowing, and reduce your risk of heart disease, diabetes, and cancer. These super berries may also help you stay slim. Their polyphenols may help keep your fat stores—and waistline—from expanding, while their high levels of vitamin C just might give your body the boost it needs to burn more fat when you exercise. Enjoy a serving or two of berries every day. One cup (145 g) of fresh berries, ½ cup (122 g) of cooked berries, ¼ cup (30 g) of dried berries, or ½ cup (120 ml) of pure, 100 percent berry juice all count as a serving.

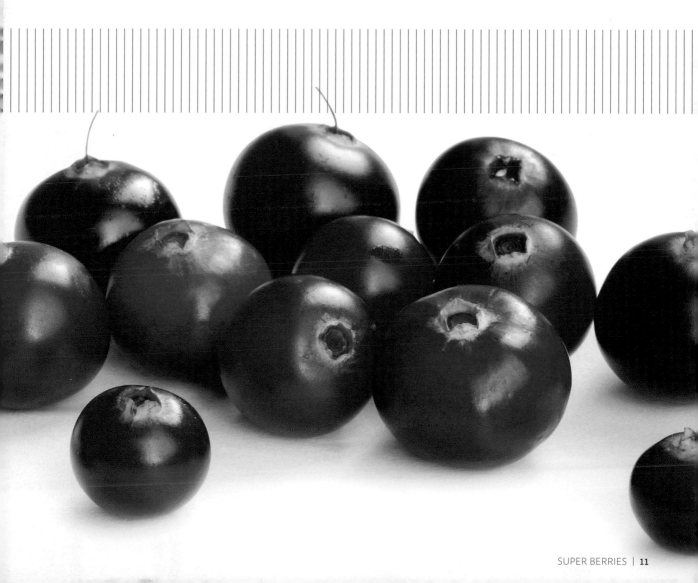

AÇAI BERRY
Antiaging Super Berry

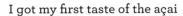

SPOTLIGHT: ANTHOCYANINS

Anthocyanins are the pigments that give plants their red, blue, and purple color. These powerful phytochemicals help prevent cell damage, reduce inflammation, and are especially known for their protective effect on the heart and brain. Foods rich in anthocyanins include all types of berries, apples, red cabbage, and red grapes.

I got my first taste of the açai (ah-sigh-ee) berry several years ago when I ordered a Brazilian breakfast bowl from the menu at my local yoga studio. The media was buzzing over the purported health benefits of this little berry, and although I could hardly pronounce its name, I decided to give it a try. I was certainly sold on the taste (who wouldn't love a combination of berries, granola, and banana?), but when it came to the health claims surrounding açai berries, had I just fallen for the hype? Not entirely. It turns out this popular super berry just might give your diet—and health—a super boost.

Super Berry of the Amazon

Native to South America, açai berries are the small, dark purple berries of tall palm trees (*Euterpe oleracea*) of the Amazon. The discovery of their numerous health-promoting compounds has led to their exploding popularity in the United States and around the world. These little berries boast an impressive nutrient profile, including nineteen amino acids, trace minerals, and beneficial fatty acids

like oleic acid, a mono-unsaturated fat also found in heart-healthy avocados and olives. But what elevates açai berries to superfood status is this: they rank among the highest of all fruits for their remarkable levels of cell-protecting antioxidants. Indeed, açai berries are rich in numerous phytochemicals—like anthocyanins, proanthocyanidins, and other flavonoids—the likely powerhouses behind their ability to slow aging, boost immunity, and protect against chronic disease.

Heart-Healthy Super Fruit with Cancer-Fighting Potential

Açai berries are good for the heart. Their anthocyanins appear to reduce inflammation in blood vessels, act as natural vasodilators (they help relax and widen the blood vessels), and lower cholesterol and triglyceride levels—all important factors in heart disease. And the protective effects of their compounds may even extend beyond the heart. In a small-scale pilot study published in *Nutrition*

Journal in May 2011, researchers looked at the effects of açai berries on various markers for heart disease and diabetes in overweight adults. After a month of consuming 100 grams (about 3½ ounces) of açai pulp twice daily, subjects experienced not only decreases in total and LDL ("bad") cholesterol levels, but also a reduced rise in blood sugars following meals and decreases in both fasting blood sugar and insulin levels—important factors in diabetes.

The high flavonoid content of açai berries may also help fight cancer. In a 2006 study conducted at the University of Florida, researchers found that extracts of açai berries triggered the self-destruction of leukemia cells, reducing their proliferation from 86 to 56 percent. Although researchers aren't sure whether the results from a test tube study can be translated directly to humans, the findings are certainly impressive enough to warrant further research on this super berry's cancer-fighting potential.

Antiaging Berry for Brains and Beauty

Açai berries are often touted as an antiaging food, and they gained much press and popularity when Nicholas Perricone, M.D., F.A.C.N., included them on his top ten list of superfoods on *Oprah* back in 2005. Studies have shown that açai berries help reduce inflammation in the brain, protect brain cells, and lower the risk of developing age-related neurological diseases like Alzheimer's and Parkinson's disease. And in addition to açai berries' fighting inflammation inside the body, the beneficial effects of their compounds may also be seen outside the body on your largest organ—your skin. Açai berries boost antioxidant levels in the skin and may help treat age-related skin concerns like hyperpigmentation. Whether eaten or used in topical preparations, these super berries may be just what you need to get your skin glowing.

PUTTING IT INTO PRACTICE

The açai berry itself is rare to find outside of South America, but its products—including bottled juices and smoothies, dried powders, frozen pulps, and sorbets—are widely available in supermarkets and health food stores. I recommend buying pure, unsweetened frozen pulps and dried powders for use at home. Although mildly tart in flavor, they make excellent additions to dishes that combine sweeter fruits like blueberries, sweet cherries, bananas, or dates. Simply add a 3½-ounce (100 g) pouch of frozen pulp or a tablespoon (15 g) or two of dried powder to freshly pressed juices, blended smoothies, cereals, or desserts for an instant nutrient infusion—it's that easy. Ready-to-drink bottled juices and smoothies may be okay, too, but they are often mixed with cheaper juices and added sugar, so be sure to read food labels before purchasing.

BERRY LAVENDER ICE CREAM

||||||||||||||||||||||||||||||||||||||||

SUPERFOOD KITCHEN TIP: SOAKING NUTS AND SEEDS

Some recipes recommend soaking nuts and seeds to improve their texture and make them easier to process. Soaking also helps release their enzyme inhibitors (compounds that keep them from sprouting prematurely), which may improve their digestion and enhance nutrient absorption. To soak, simply measure out the required portion of nuts or seeds and place in a glass bowl with at least double the amount of water (for example, 1 cup [145 g] of nuts with at least 2 cups [475 ml] of water). Cover the bowl with a lid or kitchen towel and soak for the length of time indicated by the recipe. When soaking is complete, discard the soaking water and rinse the nuts or seeds well in a colander or strainer. You can use them immediately or refrigerate in a tightly lidded container for up to three days.

A few summers ago, I tried a sample of an out-of-this-world wild berry and lavender ice cream, and I was determined to come up with my own nondairy version. When I discovered edible lavender buds at my local natural food store, I knew it was time to experiment. The result is a rich and creamy cashew-based ice cream combined with the sweetness of antioxidant-rich berries and subtle hint of stress-relieving lavender. If you can't find edible lavender buds in your market, no worries; simply leave them out and enjoy the creamy cashew and berry blend alone.

1 cup (145 g) raw cashews, soaked for 1 to 2 hours

½ cup (120 ml) water

¼ cup (80 g) agave syrup

¼ cup (55 g) coconut oil

1 packet (3½ ounces [100 g]) frozen açai berry pulp

½ cup (75 g) fresh or frozen blueberries

1 tablespoon (15 g) edible lavender, pulverized

½ vanilla bean, scraped, or ½ teaspoon pure vanilla extract

Pinch of sea salt

Yield: 4 servings

Drain and rinse the cashews. Blend the cashews, water, agave syrup, and coconut oil in a high-speed blender until smooth and creamy. Add the açai berries and blueberries and blend until well combined. Add the lavender, scraped vanilla bean, and sea salt and blend a final time until the mixture is smooth. Pour into an ice-cream maker and process per the manufacturer's instructions. Transfer to a tightly lidded container and freeze. If you do not have an ice-cream maker, simply pour the mixture into a tightly lidded container and freeze.

Keep frozen. Let stand at room temperature for a few minutes before serving to soften.

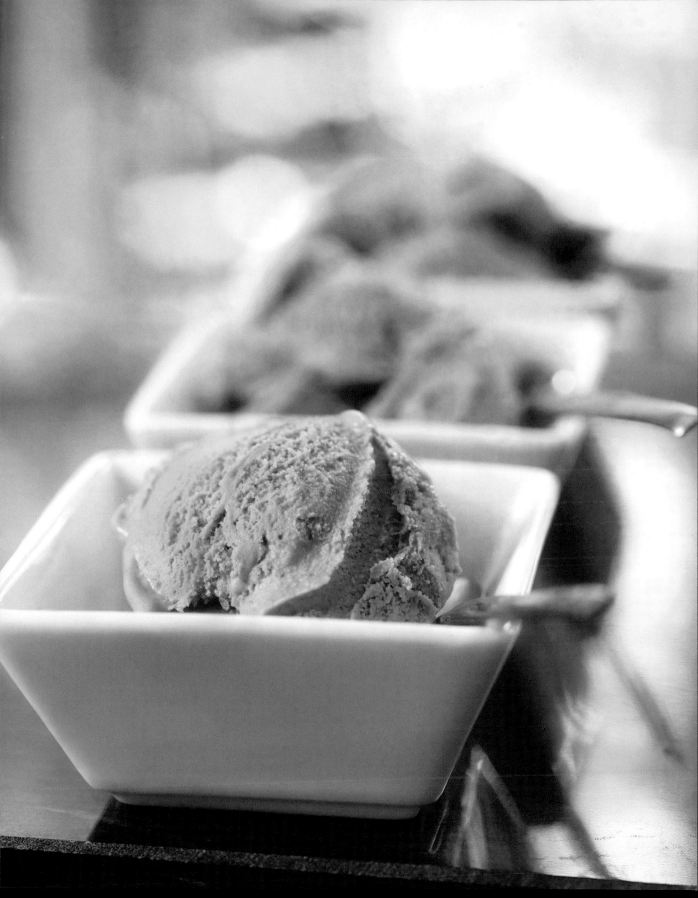

BLUEBERRY

Brain-Boosting Super Berry

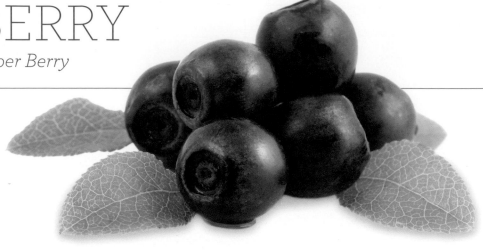

DID YOU KNOW?

Blueberries may be just as effective as cranberries in preventing urinary tract infections. Both berries contain similar compounds that prevent harmful bacteria from adhering to the bladder wall. So if the pungent taste of pure cranberry juice turns you off, try drinking pure blueberry juice or tossing a cup or more of fresh or frozen blueberries into your next smoothie for their infection-fighting power.

Annual trips to local blueberry farms were highlights of childhood summers growing up in New England. My family would pick bushels and bushels of blueberries that my mother would incorporate into at least a dozen different dishes ranging from pies and muffins to sauces and jams. And there was no shortage of blueberries in the winter, as our freezer was nearly always overflowing with bags of frozen berries from our summer harvest. Although I've always had an affinity for blueberries, little did I know just how amazing these "blue dynamos" (as they are sometimes called) really were. Native to North America, blueberries (of the *Vaccinium* genus) may not have the same allure of an exotic berry like açai, but they are just as worthy of the superfood spotlight. Ranking among the highest of all fruits for their impressive levels of antioxidants, blueberries are one of the top health-promoting superfoods in the world.

All-American Super Berry

Blueberries are good source of several important nutrients, including energy-boosting manganese, dietary fiber (around 4 grams per cup), and bone-building vitamin K, which is more commonly found in green leafy vegetables. In fact, 1 cup (145 g) of blueberries boasts nearly 30 micrograms of vitamin K—25 to 30 percent of your daily needs. But what makes the blueberry stand out is its abundance of free radical–fighting antioxidants like anthocyanins and proanthocyanidins—the same flavonoids found in açai berries. These polyphenols are potent compounds that make the blueberry an age-proofing, brain-boosting, and chronic disease–fighting superstar.

"Blue Dynamos" Boost Brain Power

A blueberry-rich diet may improve motor skills (like balance and coordination) and cognition (yes, you can improve memory and learning). Blueberries may also lower your risk of developing age-related conditions like Alzheimer's disease and dementia. It seems that the polyphenols in blueberries accumulate in areas of the brain involved in memory and learning, where they protect your brain cells from oxidative damage, improve communication between those cells, and reduce inflammation.

Indeed, blueberries just might be the fountain of youth for an aging brain. In a study published in 2011, researchers at the University of Houston found that rats following a one- or two-month blueberry-enriched diet had better memory scores than those on a nutritionally complete control diet. In fact, researchers found that the short-term addition of blueberries to the diet not only prevented memory impairment but reversed it.

Triple Threat: Blueberries Fight Cancer, Heart Disease, and Diabetes

Not only do the polyphenols in blueberries give your brain a boost, they also help fight chronic disease. Polyphenol-rich blueberries appear to inhibit the growth and proliferation of certain cancer cells, including those of the mouth, prostate, breast, cervix, and colon. A diet that includes blueberries may also help lower blood pressure and cholesterol and improve insulin sensitivity—the latter of which means your body can better regulate blood sugar levels. In a study published in the *American Journal of Clinical Nutrition* in 2012, researchers at the Harvard School of Public Health found that individuals who consumed two or more weekly servings of anthocyanin-rich foods, particularly blueberries, reduced their risk of diabetes by 23 percent compared to those who consumed less than one serving per month.

So adding just 2 or more cups (290 g or more) of blueberries to your diet each week may slash your diabetes risk by nearly a quarter.

PUTTING IT INTO PRACTICE

Fresh blueberries are in season during the summer months—typically from April to October, depending on where you live in North America—and picking your own berries or buying locally during their peak season is one of the best ways to enjoy them. Fresh berries should be plump, firm, and coated with a white protective powder known as their bloom. For optimal freshness, store blueberries in the refrigerator and wash just prior to use. If you plan ahead, you can freeze the berries from your summer harvest for use during the cold winter months. However, packaged frozen berries—preferably those that are organic and unsweetened—are also highly convenient.

Fresh blueberries can be enjoyed alone or tossed into green salads, fruit salads, smoothies, and warm bowls of rolled oats, amaranth, or quinoa. They also make nice additions to baked goods like home-made pancakes, waffles, and muffins. When blueberries are out of season, try adding a cup (155 g) or more of frozen berries to your smoothies for an antioxidant boost. These sweet berries blend well with mildly tart açai berries and greens like spinach, kale, and dandelion greens—all superfoods in their own right.

BLUEBERRY OATMEAL BOWL

SUPERFOOD KITCHEN TIP: HOLD THE MILK

If you want to get a boost of antioxidants from blueberries, you may need to ditch the dairy. In a study published in 2009, researchers found that when subjects consumed 200 grams (about 7 ounces) of blueberries with water, antioxidant absorption and capacity (ability to scavenge free radicals) increased. But when they consumed the same amount of blueberries with whole milk, no such increases were seen. It appears that the antioxidants in blueberries have an affinity for milk proteins, thus reducing their antioxidant activity when the two foods are eaten together. So hold the milk and prepare your berry oatmeal bowls (and other berry-based dishes) with plain water or nondairy milk—like coconut or almond milk—for an antioxidant boost.

I like to think of this oatmeal bowl as the all-American version of the Brazilian breakfast bowl. It combines heart-healthy rolled oats with a generous serving—not just a sprinkle—of high-antioxidant blueberries. Topped with omega-3 fatty acid–rich walnuts and potassium-rich banana slices, this dish is a simple and nutritious way to start your day.

1½ cups (355 ml) water
Pinch of sea salt
¾ cup (60 g) rolled oats
1 cup (145 g) blueberries
¼ teaspoon pure vanilla extract
½ medium-size banana, sliced
¼ cup (30 g) raw walnuts, chopped
Pure maple syrup, to serve (optional)

Bring the water and salt to a boil in a small saucepan. Stir in the oats and reduce the heat. Simmer uncovered, stirring occasionally, until the oats are tender, about 10 minutes. Remove from the heat and stir in the blueberries and vanilla extract. Transfer to a bowl and top with the sliced banana and walnuts. Drizzle with maple syrup, if desired. Serve warm.

Note: This recipe is gluten free if you choose to use gluten-free rolled oats. Although traditional oats don't contain wheat, rye, or barley (all of which contain gluten), they may become contaminated with these gluten-containing grains during cultivation and processing. For this reason, if you are following a gluten-free diet, consume only oats labeled "gluten free."

Yield: 2 servings

   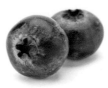

18 | POWERFUL PLANT-BASED SUPERFOODS

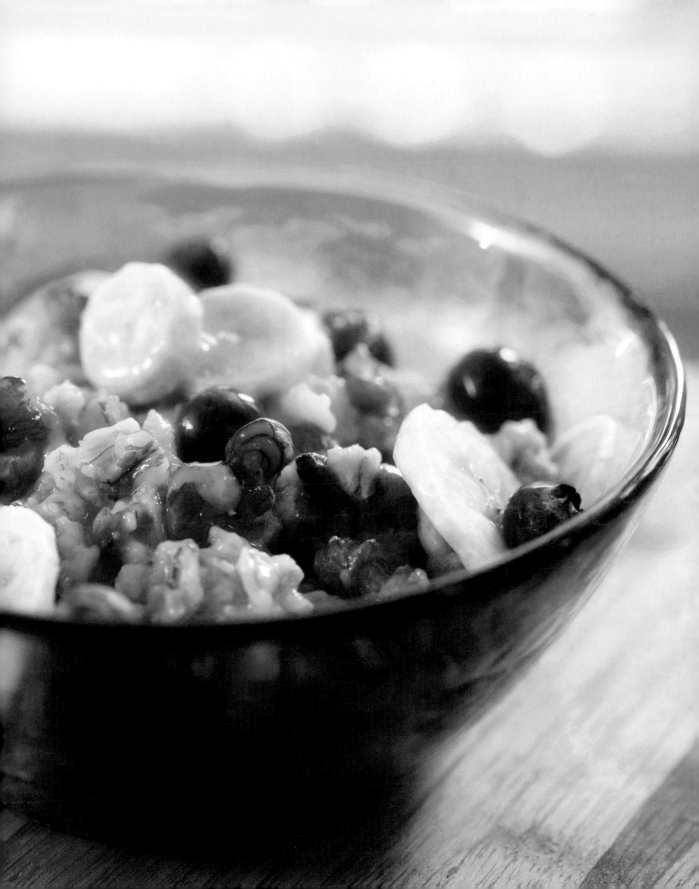

CAMU CAMU BERRY

Vitamin C–Rich Super Berry

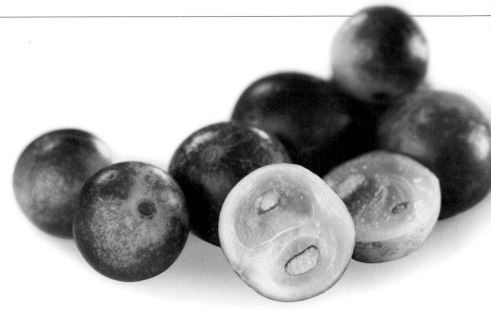

Vitamin C won't prevent a cold, but it can help treat it. Researchers have found that supplementing with vitamin C—as little as 200 milligrams daily—may shorten the duration and lessen the severity of the common cold. But here's the caveat: you need to be consuming that amount on a daily basis; simply increasing your intake of vitamin C after your cold has already started seems to have little to no effect. So eat plenty of vitamin C–rich foods every day, especially during cold and flu season, to keep your defenses strong. Two cups (290 g) of strawberries, 1 cup (150 g) of chopped red bell peppers, 2 large oranges, or slightly less than ¼ teaspoon of camu camu powder all contain around 200 milligrams of vitamin C.

Only recently have I started experimenting with the exotic camu camu berry. Although I frequently consume the berries that grow in my own backyard, New York's long winter months often leave me looking for options that extend beyond the region. So in addition to buying bags of unsweetened, frozen organic berries, I also reach for the dried powders and frozen pulps of exotic berries for both diversity and nutrition. And when I discovered just how high in vitamin C the camu camu berry was, I thought it would make an exceptional addition to the diet—especially during the winter months, when cold and flu season is at its peak. As it turns out, this tangy berry might be just what you need to give your body an antioxidant boost during the winter season—and all year long.

Camu Camu Berries Are Nature's Vitamin C

Camu camu berries are small, red berries that grow on tropical bushes (*Myrciaria dubia*) in the flooded lowlands of the Amazon rain forest. Traditionally, these berries have been used to support the immune system; fight cold and flu viruses; maintain healthy eyes, gums, and skin; and strengthen body tissues like collagen, tendons, and ligaments.

Although there is little published research on the health benefits of this emerging super berry, we do know that it is an exceptionally good source of vitamin C, an essential water-soluble vitamin that assists in the growth and repair of all body tissues. This antioxidant helps produce collagen, a structural component of the skin, blood vessels, tendons, ligaments, and bones; norepinephrine, a chemical that supports brain function; and carnitine, a compound that helps the body turn fat into energy. Vitamin C is a potent antioxidant through which even small amounts can combat the damaging effects of oxidative stress on the body—and the camu camu berry is reported to be one of the richest known sources of vitamin C in the world. One teaspoon of camu camu powder contains more than 1,000 percent of your daily vitamin C needs.

Inflammation-Fighting Berry of the Amazon

Camu camu berries appear to have strong antioxidant and inflammation-fighting activities. In a study published in 2008 in the *Journal of Cardiology*, researchers tested the effects of camu camu juice on various markers of inflammation and oxidative stress in male smokers. Twenty subjects were given a daily dose of either 1,050 milligrams of vitamin C or 70 milliliters (about 2 ounces, or ¼ cup) of camu camu juice, which contained 1,050 milligrams of vitamin C. After seven days, researchers found that although the vitamin C supplement had no effect on inflammatory markers, treatment with camu camu juice significantly decreased those markers. The findings suggested that in addition to vitamin C—or perhaps in spite of it—there are other nutrients in these berries that help exert its protective effects.

Camu camu berries appear to be a good source of polyphenols, including ellagic acid and flavonoids like anthocyanin, which may help improve lipid profiles (including cholesterol and triglyceride levels) and promote heart health. They also contain smaller amounts of cancer-fighting carotenoids with the majority—45 to 55 percent—in the form of lutein, which helps prevent age-related eye diseases like cataracts and macular degeneration.

PUTTING IT INTO PRACTICE

Fresh camu camu berries are hard to find outside of South America, but bottled juices and dried powders are becoming increasingly available at supermarkets and health food stores. The tart and tangy berry powder can be added in small amounts—about ¼ to 1 teaspoon—to your favorite freshly pressed juices, blended smoothies, and salad dressings for a boost of vitamin C and other antioxidants. If you decide to purchase camu camu juice, read food labels. Many juices contain a blend of tart camu camu berries and cheaper, sweeter juices. Although they make the juice more palatable, they often deliver more sugar and fewer of camu camu berry's health-promoting nutrients.

SPINACH AND STRAWBERRY SALAD WITH ORANGE CAMU DRESSING

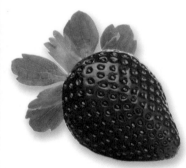

This simple salad incorporates several well-matched power foods. One bunch of spinach has nearly 10 grams of blood-building iron— 55 to 125 percent of your daily needs—and the vitamin C in the strawberries, orange juice, and camu camu powder enhances your body's ability to absorb that iron. Your body will also get a nice boost of inflammation-fighting omega-3 fatty acids from the addition of maple-glazed walnuts whose sweet flavor are a nice complement to the tart and tangy dressing. Enjoy this salad in the spring—when spinach and strawberries are in season—or any time of year.

For the Maple-Glazed Walnuts:

½	cup (60 g) raw walnuts, chopped
1	tablespoon (20 g) pure maple syrup
	Pinch of sea salt

For the Dressing:

1	tablespoon (15 ml) balsamic vinegar
1	teaspoon pure maple syrup
1	small clove garlic, crushed
½	teaspoon orange zest
¼	teaspoon camu camu powder
3	tablespoons (45 ml) extra-virgin olive oil
	Sea salt and freshly ground pepper, to taste

For the Salad:

6 to 8	cups (180 to 240 g) loosely packed fresh spinach
2	cups (340 g) hulled and sliced fresh strawberries

Yield: 4 to 6 servings

To make the maple-glazed walnuts: Preheat the oven to 325°F (170°C, or gas mark 3). Combine the walnuts, maple syrup, and sea salt in a small bowl. Spread on a rimmed baking sheet and toast on the center rack of oven for about 10 minutes, stirring occasionally. The nuts will turn golden brown when done. Let cool completely before adding to the salad.

To make the dressing: Combine the vinegar, maple syrup, garlic, orange zest, and camu camu powder. Whisk in the olive oil and season with salt and freshly ground pepper, to taste.

To make the salad: Place the spinach, strawberries, and cooled maple-glazed walnuts in a large serving bowl. Toss gently with the dressing until well coated.

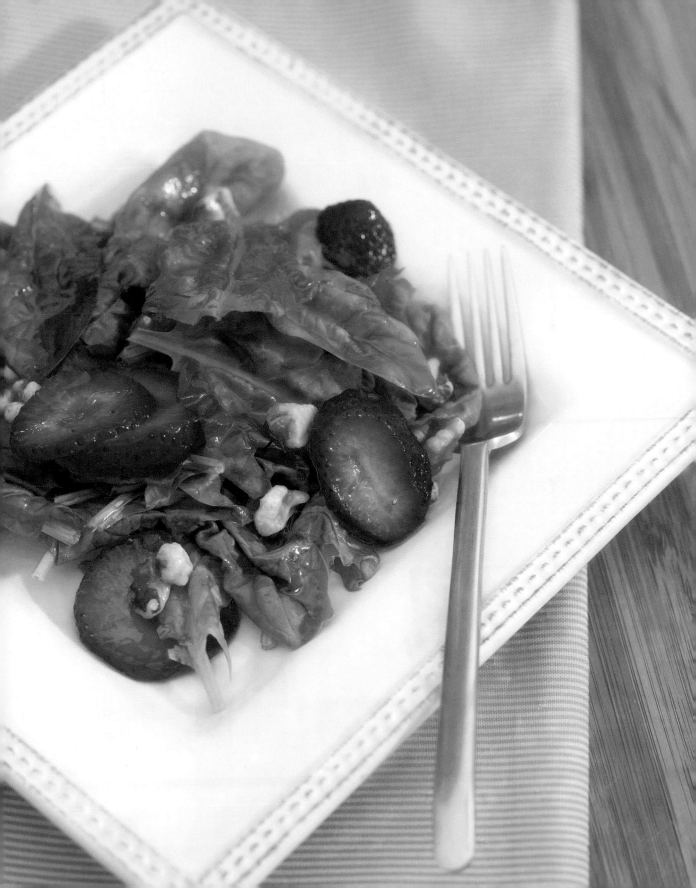

CRANBERRY

Infection-Fighting Super Berry

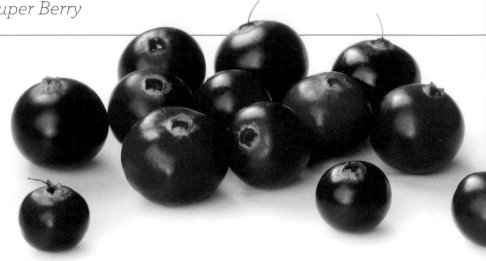

DID YOU KNOW?

You can get an antioxidant boost from all forms of cranberries. Researchers have found that 8 ounces (235 ml) of 25 percent cranberry juice cocktail, 1½ cups (150 g) of fresh or frozen cranberries, 1 ounce (28 g) of dried cranberries, and ½ cup (139 g) of cranberry sauce all have the same level of antioxidants—and infection-fighting power. So eat—and drink—up for good health!

SPOTLIGHT: ELLAGIC ACID

Ellagic acid is a polyphenol that has potent antioxidant activity. It appears to play an important role in heart disease but is probably best known for its cancer-fighting potential. Cell studies have found that ellagic acid may induce cell death in cancer cells and help eliminate cancer-causing substances from the body. Good sources of ellagic acid include berries like cranberries, strawberries, and raspberries; pomegranates; and nuts like walnuts and pecans.

Cranberries are often associated with Thanksgiving—at least for those of us living in the United States. But this super berry can—and should—be enjoyed year-round. One of three commercially grown fruits native to North America (along with blueberries and Concord grapes), cranberries are the small, red berries of low-growing, woody perennial plants (*Vaccinium macrocarpon*) that are cultivated on more than 40,000 acres across the northern United States and Canada. The cranberry has a long history of use as food and medicine, and with research documenting its beneficial roles in everything from heart disease and cancer to urinary tract infections and ulcers, this little red berry is a modern-day power food.

The Berry with Bacteria-Blocking Power

Cranberries are an infection-fighting super berry. They are an excellent source of a group of flavonoids called proanthocyanidins, which are thought to be the force behind this berry's unique ability to prevent bacterial infections. Rather than destroy harmful bacteria, these beneficial compounds prevent bacteria from adhering to the walls of various tissues and organs like the bladder, stomach, teeth, and gums.

Indeed, eating cranberries may decrease your risk of urinary tract infections. The proanthocyanidins in these super berries help keep bacteria like *Escherichia coli* from sticking to the bladder walls—and they even appear to act on strains of bacteria that are resistant to traditional antibiotic treatments. The beneficial effects of cranberries appear to be greatest in women with recurrent urinary tract infections, and researchers have found that drinking just one cup (235 ml) of cranberry juice is enough to keep harmful bacteria at bay for up to ten hours.

The infection-fighting power of the cranberry is not limited to the bladder. In the mouth, the beneficial proanthocyanidins prevent bacteria from adhering to the teeth and gums, where they can cause gum disease and cavities. And in the stomach, these beneficial compounds keep *Helicobacter pylori*, a bacterium whose presence in the gut is known to be a major risk factor for both ulcers and stomach cancer, from adhering to the stomach wall.

In a study published in 2007, researchers looked at the effects of cranberry juice on patients with *H. pylori* infections. In conjunction with antibiotic treatment, they found that the eradication rate of *H. pylori* was greater in females receiving 250 milliliters (about 8½ ounces) of cranberry juice twice daily compared to those who received a placebo beverage and antibiotics or antibiotics alone.

Cranberries Keep the Heart Healthy and Fight Cancer

The combination of polyphenols in cranberries, including flavonoids like proanthocyanidins and nonflavonoids like ellagic acid, gives this little berry its strong antioxidant and anti-inflammatory properties. Cranberries may help reduce total and LDL ("bad") cholesterol levels, improve HDL ("good") cholesterol levels, and prevent atherosclerosis (hardening of the arteries)—all important factors in heart disease. And when it comes to cancer, researchers have found that cranberry extracts can reduce the growth and proliferation of certain cancer cells, including those of the breast, colon, lung, and prostate.

PUTTING IT INTO PRACTICE

Cranberries are harvested between September and October in North America, and fresh berries are typically available from early fall through December. When fresh cranberries are not in season, look for unsweetened, frozen, or dried cranberries in your supermarket or health food store. Although fresh and frozen berries are generally too tart to be consumed alone, they make great additions to smoothies that include sweeter fruits and can be heated and cooked into sauces. Dried cranberries can be sprinkled onto warm bowls of oats, amaranth, or quinoa; baked into muffins and breads; or tossed onto green salads and steamed vegetables.

Unsweetened and sweetened cranberry juices, the latter of which is often called cranberry juice cocktail, are other options for getting an antioxidant boost of this superfood. However, cranberry juice cocktail packs a whopping 30 grams of sugar per cup, so I don't recommend it. Instead, trying putting a splash—around 2 ounces or ¼ cup (60 ml)—of 100 percent pure, unsweetened cranberry juice into a freshly pressed juice, smoothie, or glass of sparkling water for an antioxidant-rich beverage. You will get a similar dose of beneficial antioxidants with far less sugar—4 to 8 grams.

CRANBERRY-BLUEBERRY SAUCE

This thick and tart-sweet cranberry sauce is a modified version of the recipe my mom made when I was growing up. By combining tart cranberries with sweet blueberries, I was able to use less than half the amount of sugar originally used in this recipe, while substituting pure, mineral-rich maple syrup for brown and white sugars. Enjoy this zesty sauce alone as a side dish or topped on warm bowls of cereal, whole-grain toast, sweet potatoes, or winter squash.

4 cups (400 g) fresh or frozen cranberries

2 cups (290 g) fresh or frozen blueberries

½ cup (160 g) pure maple syrup

3 tablespoons (45 ml) freshly squeezed orange juice

1 teaspoon orange zest
Pinch of ground cinnamon

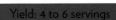
Yield: 4 to 6 servings

Combine the cranberries and blueberries, maple syrup, and orange juice in a large saucepan. Bring to a boil, reduce the heat, and simmer uncovered, stirring occasionally, until the berries burst, 8 to 10 minutes (longer for frozen berries and shorter for fresh). Remove from the heat, add the orange zest and cinnamon, and stir to combine. The sauce will thicken as it cools. Let cool at room temperature before serving. Refrigerate if preparing in advance.

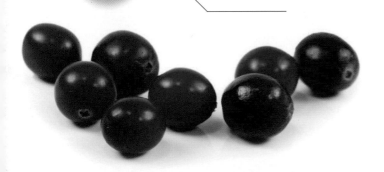

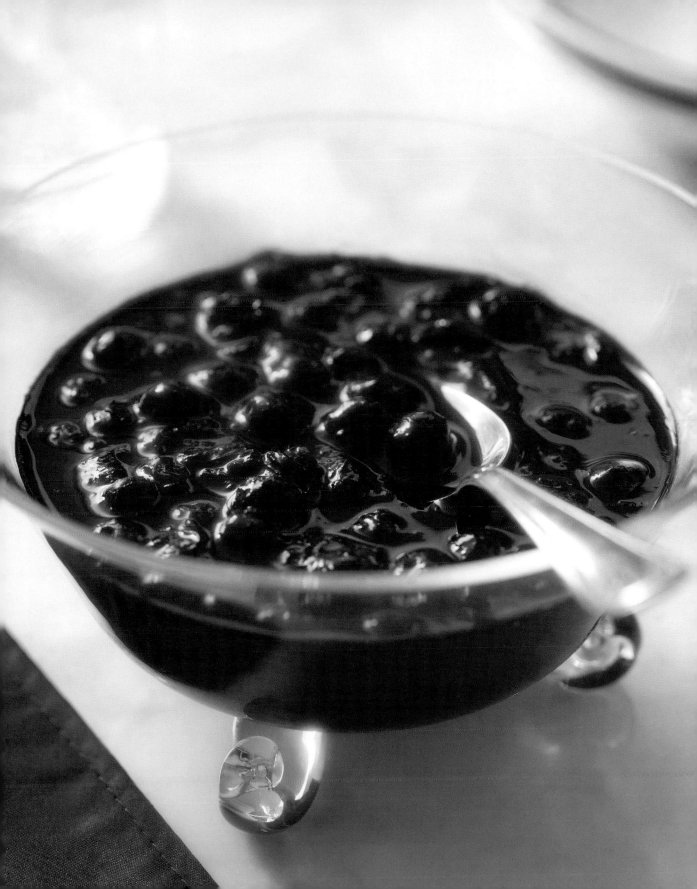

GOJI BERRY
Super Berry for Vitality

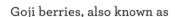

DID YOU KNOW?

You can eat your sunscreen (well, sort of). Topical sunscreens protect your skin from sun damage, such as wrinkles, sun spots, and skin cancer. And eating antioxidant-rich foods—like goji berries—can also help boost your skin's defenses. In a study published in 2010, researchers at the University of Sydney found that when mice drank 5 percent goji berry juice, the antioxidant activity in their skin increased and the damaging effects of exposure to ultraviolet rays—including inflammation from sunburn—were reduced. In addition to goji berries, quercetin-rich apples and onions, curcumin-packed turmeric, selenium-rich Brazil nuts, and resveratrol-containing red wine and grapes all have sun- and skin-protecting antioxidants.

Goji berries, also known as wolfberries, are the bright red-orange berries from a deciduous shrub (*Lycium barbarum*) that is native to China. They have been used for thousands of years to promote health and longevity. In fact, traditional Chinese medicine practitioners have long used them to treat diabetes and high blood pressure; maintain eye health; nourish the liver and kidneys; and enhance energy, stamina, and sexual performance. Today, goji berries are enjoying exploding popularity due to similar modern-day claims. And, indeed, a growing body of research is discovering that this super berry just might give your body, health, and even your sex life a super boost.

Packed with Immune-Supporting and Cancer-Fighting Complexes

Goji berries are a rich source of vitamins C and E and carotenoids like beta-carotene and lycopene. They even contain small amounts of beneficial polyphenols like flavonoids and ellagic acid. But probably one of the most important and active constituents of goji berries are the *Lycium barbarum* polysaccharide-protein complexes, also known as LBP. Consisting of long chains of sugars and amino acids, these complexes have potent antioxidant, anti-inflammatory, and antiaging properties. They help protect the organs of the body—including the eyes, brain, and liver—from the damaging effects of oxidative stress. And they also appear to play an important role in immune function.

The LBP complexes are powerful immune boosters that may help increase the activity of the body's white blood cells, including the macrophages, T cells, and natural killer cells—all of which protect the body from infection and foreign invaders. In fact, researchers have found that LBP extracts of goji berries—in addition to other active compounds within the berry—can actually trigger the self-destruction of leukemia and breast, prostate, colon, and liver cancer cells, among others.

Goji: The Go-to Berry for a Metabolism Boost

Goji berries have long been used to promote vitality, energy, and stamina. And in some human studies, subjects consuming goji berries and their juices have reported better digestion, less fatigue and stress, and an improved sense of well-being. Several animal studies suggest that goji berries may help increase metabolism, improve energy levels, and even reduce body weight gains.

In a study published in 2011 in the *Journal of the American College of Nutrition*, researchers looked at the effects of goji berries in healthy overweight adults in two small randomized, double-blind, placebo-controlled studies. They found that subjects who consumed a single dose of 30, 60, or 120 milliliters—about 1, 2, and 4 ounces, respectively—of a goji berry–based juice boosted their metabolic rate after meals by as much as 10 percent compared to the placebo group. And the effects appeared to be dose dependent, meaning that the more goji berry juice they consumed—up to 120 milliliters (4 ounces, or ½ cup)—the better the results. In addition, researchers found that subjects who consumed 120 milliliters of goji berry juice over a fourteen-day period experienced reductions in their waist circumference.

Libido-Boosting Berry

Goji berries also have a long history of use for enhancing sexual performance and fertility. A few animal studies have found that extracts of LBP from goji berries—the same complexes that help support immune function—may also boost libido, improve sexual performance, increase sperm quantity and motility, and exert a protective effect on male reproductive organs. In a study published in 2012, researchers from China looked at the effects of goji berries on sexual performance in rats fed daily extracts of LBP over a twenty-one-day period. They found that rats consuming LBP extracts experienced enhanced sexual behavior, including improved sexual interest, performance, and increased frequency of ejaculation, among other factors. The extracts also helped prevent low sex drive following the administration of certain steroids likely to cause sexual inhibition. So if you are looking to give your sex life a boost, goji berries may be a welcome addition in the kitchen—and bedroom.

PUTTING IT INTO PRACTICE

You can find goji berries in most supermarkets and health food stores in the form of whole dried berries, dried powders, and juices. I recommend dried goji berries over powders or juices. In addition to their beneficial antioxidants, a 2-ounce (55 g) serving of these mildly sweet berries provides about 8 grams of protein (more than an egg) and 6 grams of dietary fiber—two nutrients you won't find in a bottled juice or powder.

The soft and chewy, raisinlike texture of dried goji berries make them perfect for snacking on alone or blending into soups and smoothies. They also make a great addition to homemade trail mixes (my favorite combination is a simple mix of goji berries, cashews, pumpkin seeds, and cacao nibs), hot and cold cereals, and green salads.

CARROT-GOJI BERRY SOUP

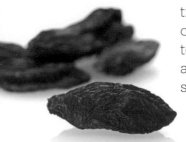

When I was living and working in Washington, D.C., I often made treks to my P Street Whole Foods Market to pick up my favorite carrot-ginger soup. Little did I realize just how simple this soup was to create at home—and just how tasty it would be with one small addition: goji berries. The carrots and goji berries in this creamy soup are packed with immune-boosting vitamins A and C and add a hint of sweetness to this dish, while freshly grated ginger gives it an inflammation-fighting and subtly spicy boost.

1 tablespoon (14 g) coconut oil

1 medium-size onion, chopped

1 tablespoon (8 g) grated fresh ginger

8 to 10 medium-size carrots, peeled and sliced thinly

6 cups (1.4 L) vegetable stock

½ cup (45 g) dried goji berries
Sea salt and freshly-ground pepper, to taste

Yield: 6 to 8 servings

Warm the coconut oil in a large pot over medium heat. Add the onion and ginger and sauté until the onion is soft, about 3 minutes. Add the carrots and vegetable stock. Bring to a boil, reduce the heat, and simmer, covered, until the carrots are soft, about 30 minutes. Remove from the heat and add the goji berries and salt and pepper, to taste. Using an immersion blender, purée the soup until it is smooth. (If you do not have an immersion blender, allow the soup to cool, purée in small batches in a high-speed blender, and return to the stockpot.) Cover the soup and warm over low heat until ready to serve. Individual bowls of soup can be garnished with a sprinkle of whole, dried goji berries.

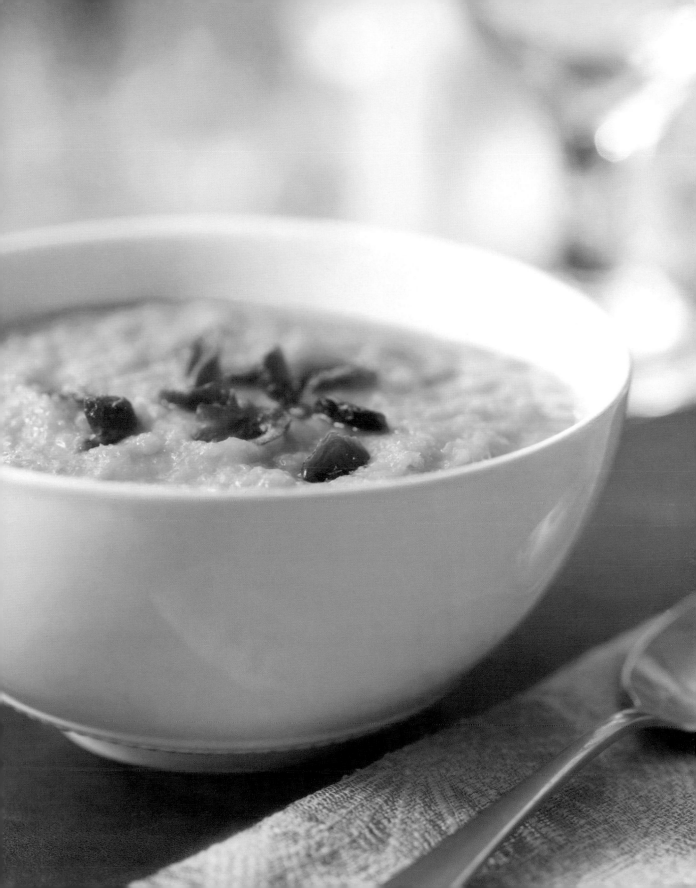

GOLDENBERRY
Nature's Sweet-Tart Super Berry

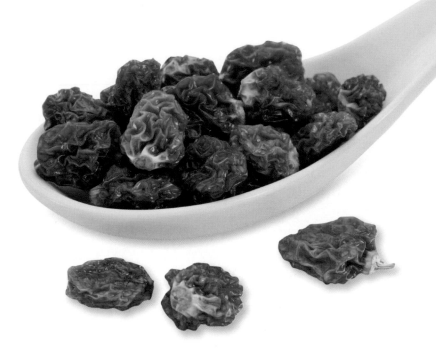

SPOTLIGHT: VITAMIN A

Vitamin A is a fat-soluble vitamin with strong antioxidant activity. It helps boost the immune system, protects vision, and plays an important role in bone growth, cell function, and reproduction. Vitamin A from plant foods is in the form of provitamin A carotenoids, which include beta-carotene, alpha-carotene, and beta-cryptoxanthin. These compounds are converted into vitamin A in the body, and good sources include leafy green vegetables like spinach and kale, as well as orange and yellow foods like carrots, sweet potatoes, cantaloupe, and—you guessed it—goldenberries.

Goldenberries, also known as Incan berries or cape gooseberries, are the yellow-orange berries of a small perennial shrub (*Physalis peruviana*) native to South America. These plants grow wild throughout various parts of the Andes and have a long history of use in folk medicine, including the treatment of cancer, hepatitis, dermatitis, asthma, malaria, rheumatism, and other conditions. Interestingly, in traditional Colombian medicine, goldenberry juice has been used as a topical eye remedy for the treatment of pterygium, a condition that can lead to vision loss and blindness. Indeed, researchers are just beginning to uncover the beneficial

nutritional and medicinal properties of this little tart berry, making it an increasingly popular fruit throughout Europe, the United States, and around the world.

Goldenberries Keep You Active and Moving

Goldenberries have been touted as a superfood for energy and weight. Back in 2011, Mehmet Oz, M.D., included goldenberries as one of "Dr. Oz's 3 Breakthrough Belly Blasters" because of its rich content of B vitamins. I don't know for sure if these little berries can blast through belly fat, but they certainly contain the nutrients you need to support energy

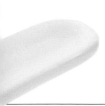

levels and reduce belly bloat.

Goldenberries' stress-reducing B-complex vitamins help support the immune system, nervous system, and adrenal glands, the latter of which helps regulate metabolism. And they are key factors in helping you unlock the energy from the food you eat—turning every meal and snack into energy your body can use.

Goldenberries are also rich in protein and fiber, both of which help slow the release of its sugars into the bloodstream, providing you with a steady supply of energy. A single ounce of dried berries (a small handful [8 g]) contains about 2 grams of protein and 3 grams of dietary fiber, the latter of which meets about 10 percent of your daily fiber needs. They help keep you fuller longer (so you are less likely to overeat) and keep the bowels moving (preventing uncomfortable stomach bloating and distention).

Active Compounds in Goldenberries May Help Fight Cancer

Goldenberries contain antioxidant and anti-inflammatory compounds that protect tissues and organs in the body from the damaging effects of free radicals and exposure to toxins. They are a good source of antioxidant vitamins C and A; in fact, a 1-ounce (28 g) serving of dried goldenberries meets nearly half of your daily vitamin A needs.

Researchers have also identfied a group of natural steroidal compounds in goldenberries called withanolides, which appear to have strong anticancer activities. In cell studies, phytochemical-rich extracts of goldenberries have been found to inhibit the growth and proliferation of certain cancers, including those of the lungs, liver, and breast. And in a study published in 2010, researchers found that a specific withanolide in goldenberries, 4beta-Hydroxywithanolide E (4beta-HWE), was able to stop the growth of lung cancer cells by damaging their genetic material and causing them to self-destruct—all without affecting healthy lung cells.

PUTTING IT INTO PRACTICE

Goldenberries can be enjoyed in both their fresh and dried forms, and although fresh berries are not common outside of South America, dried berries can be purchased at most supermarkets and health food stores. Dried goldenberries have a sweet-tart flavor and slightly tougher texture than that of a raisin. They can be enjoyed alone as a snack or mixed into homemade trail mixes, cereals, or salads. Try adding a serving of this super berry—¼ cup (30 g) dried—to your diet for a boost of cancer-fighting compounds and energy-producing B-complex vitamins.

APPLE AND FENNEL SALAD WITH GOLDENBERRIES

SUPERFOOD KITCHEN TIP: DON'T PEEL YOUR APPLES

The humble apple is an often overlooked power food that is a rich source of cancer-fighting phytochemicals. But did you know that when you peel an apple, you discard some of these important compounds? In a study published in 2008, researchers at Cornell University identified more than a dozen compounds in apple peels (including triterpenoids, flavonoids, and other phytochemicals) that can inhibit or destroy certain cancer cells. So enjoy fresh apples with their skins—and get ready to soak up their health-giving power.

One of my favorite juice combinations is fennel and apple with just a sprinkle of cinnamon on top. In this simple salad, those favorites are merged into a delicious dish that combines the bloat-reducing power of fennel with fiber-rich apples, almonds, goldenberries, and whole flaxseeds. Enjoy for breakfast—or any time of day.

2 apples, cored and sliced
1 bulb fennel, chopped
¼ cup (36 g) raw almonds
1 tablespoon (15 ml) freshly squeezed lemon juice
1 tablespoon (12 g) whole flaxseeds
¼ teaspoon ground cinnamon
½ cup (60 g) dried goldenberries

Place all the ingredients except the goldenberries in a food processor and pulse into a coarse mixture. Transfer to a bowl, stir in the goldenberries, and serve.

Yield: 2 to 3 servings

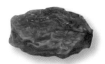
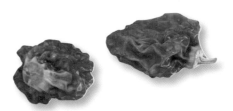

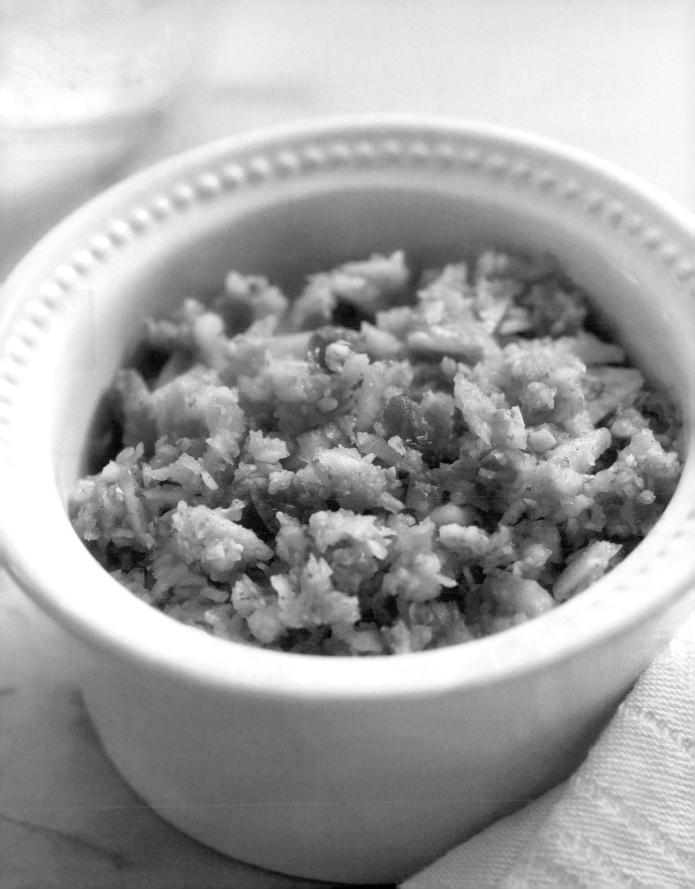

MAQUI BERRY
Super Antioxidant-Rich Berry

ⅢⅢⅢⅢⅢⅢⅢⅢⅢⅢⅢⅢⅢⅢⅢ

DID YOU KNOW?

Berries may help you stay slim. In the body, fat cells can increase in both size and number, and over time, this can lead to obesity. But several studies have found that the polyphenols in berries seem to interfere with the pathways involved in the growth and development of fat cells. In cell studies, they appear to reduce inflammation, prevent fat deposition (to keep existing fat cells from getting bigger), and inhibit the production of new fat cells (to keep them from increasing in number). Although it's hard to say whether the results of a cell study would have the same effect in the body, loading up on berries and other polyphenol-rich foods—like pomegranates, grapes, and green tea—may be good for your health and your waistline.

South American fruits are becoming increasingly popular as researchers begin to uncover their impressive levels of antioxidants and potential health benefits—and the maqui berry is no exception. Sometimes referred to as the Chilean blackberry, maqui berries are the small purple berries of the fruit-bearing shrub *Aristotelia chilensis*. It grows abundantly throughout the Patagonia region of southern Chile, where it is harvested by the indigenous Mapuche Indian tribes. Maqui berries—and their leaves—have long been used to treat conditions ranging from ulcers and diarrhea to sore throat and fever. And today, researchers are just beginning to take interest in this berry whose striking levels of antioxidants make it a superfood to watch.

Free Radical- and Fat-Fighting Fruit

In a study published in 2012, researchers at the University of Chile looked at the antioxidant levels of twenty-seven fruits produced and consumed in the south Andes region of South America. The fruits were ranked according to their oxygen radical absorbance capacity (ORAC) values, which are simply a measure of their antioxidant capacity (how well they can scavenge cell-damaging free radicals in laboratory studies). Although all berries in the study came out on top, the maqui berry ranked second among all fruits. In fact, the maqui berry had a greater ORAC score than three traditionally grown berries of the region (blueberries, raspberries, and blackberries) and one native berry of the region (murtilla berry).

Maqui berries are high in heart-healthy flavonoids, including proanthocyanidins and anthocyanins, the latter of which give these berries—as well as blueberries and açai berries—their deep purple color. Research suggests that the maqui berry may help prevent atherosclerosis and its high levels of flavonoids may help reduce inflammation in blood vessels, act as natural vasodilators (they relax and widen the blood vessels), and lower cholesterol and triglyceride levels. A few studies have even found that a main anthocyanin in the maqui berry, delphinidin-3-glucoside, may help regulate blood sugars—an important factor for those with diabetes.

Maqui berries, like other antioxidant-rich foods, may also play a future role in the management of obesity. In a study published in 2010, University of Illinois researchers looked at the effects of polyphenol-rich extracts of maqui berries and a type of South American blueberry (*Vaccinium floribundum*) on fat cells. They found that extracts of these berries reduced inflammation in fat cells and inhibited the accumulation of fat by 4 to 11 percent in mature fat cells and by 6 to 38 percent in developing fat cells.

PUTTING IT INTO PRACTICE

Maqui berry powders and juices are becoming more widely available in supermarkets and health food stores. Maqui berry powder has a mild flavor and a teaspoon or two can be easily blended into smoothies or sprinkled on warm bowls of oatmeal, amaranth, or quinoa. You can also add a splash—about 2 ounces (¼ cup [60 ml])—of 100 percent, pure maqui berry juice to your freshly pressed juices, blended smoothies, or sparkling water for an antioxidant boost.

MAQUI BERRY LIMEADE

Most of the beverages in this book yield 3 to 5 cups (700 to 1,140 ml)—enough for two 12- to 20-ounce (355 to 570 g) servings of a fresh juice or smoothie. How much liquid each recipe yields depends on the size of the fruits and vegetables used (your medium-size cucumber may be much larger than mine) and how fresh those fruits and vegetables are (more juice can be extracted from fresher fruits and veggies). But in general, you can expect two generous servings for each juice and smoothie recipe in this book. And although it is best to drink freshly pressed juices and smoothies right away, unless otherwise specified, you can store any extra in the refrigerator in a tightly lidded container (I like to use Ball mason jars) for up to twenty-four hours.

This maqui berry limeade is subtly sweet and highly refreshing. The combination of potassium- and magnesium-rich coconut water and antioxidant-rich maqui berries make it the perfect beverage for hydrating, replenishing electrolytes, and boosting antioxidants following a hard workout or on a hot summer day.

3 cups (700 ml) coconut water, chilled

Juice of 2 limes (or more for flavor)

1 tablespoon (20 g) agave syrup

1 tablespoon (8 g) maqui berry powder

Lime slices, for garnish (optional)

Blend all the ingredients in a high-speed blender. Pour over ice and garnish with a few lime slices, if desired. If making a large batch, store in a tightly lidded glass pitcher in the refrigerator for up to three days. Shake before serving, as the maqui berry powder will settle to the bottom.

Yield: 2 servings

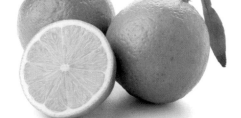

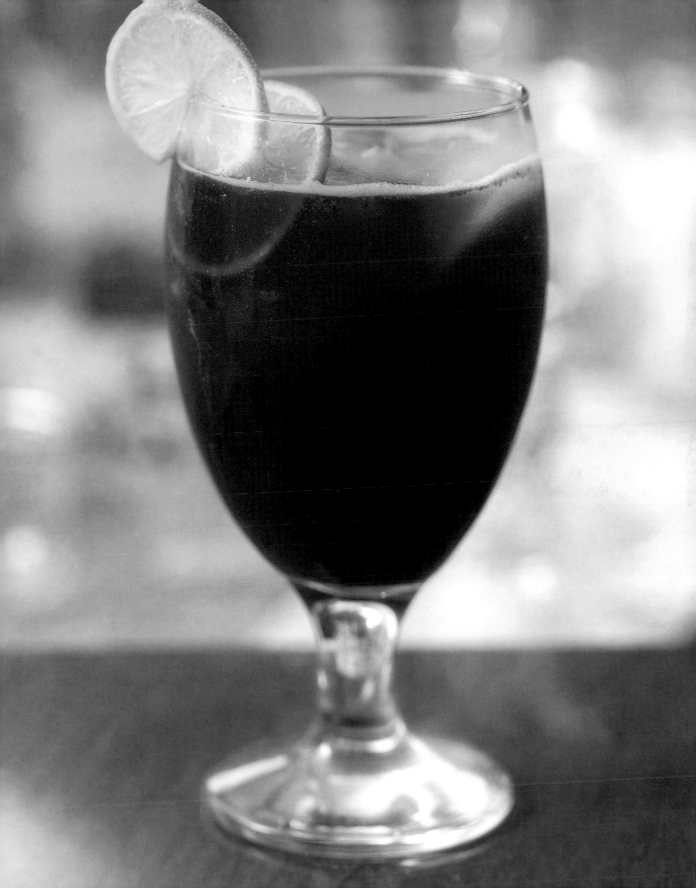

MULBERRY
Heart-Healthy Super Berry

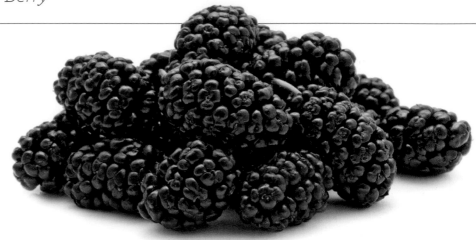

Mulberries are the berrylike fruits of the *Morus* genus of deciduous trees, of which there are an estimated twenty-four different species and one hundred known varieties.

Botanically, the mulberry is not a true berry; it is a collective fruit that is formed from a mass of flowers, like the pineapple. Mulberries are grown throughout the world, including Asia, Europe, North and South America, and Africa; I enjoy eating fresh mulberries straight from the trees here in New York.

All parts of the tree—including the leaves, bark, branches, and fruits—are high in antioxidants, and today, researchers are finding that these edible berries may play a role in promoting heart health, preventing cancer, and age-proofing your brain. Indeed, the mulberry is becoming an increasingly popular superfood for optimal health and vitality.

Super Berry for Super Heart Health

Mulberries are a rich source of heart-healthy polyphenols, including resveratrol, an antioxidant found in grapes and other berries, and flavonoids like anthocyanins and quercetin. In fact, like the açai berry, the majority of beneficial polyphenols in mulberries—particularly black mulberries (*Morus nigra*)—are anthocyanins, which not only give the fresh berry its dark color but also help keep your blood vessels healthy. These compounds reduce inflammation in blood vessels, act as natural vasodilators (they help relax and widen the blood vessels), and may lower your risk of atherosclerosis (hardening of the arteries). The anthocyanin-rich extracts from mulberries, along with other polyphenols, may also help lower blood cholesterol and triglyceride levels—two important markers for heart disease.

In a study published in 2010, researchers looked at the effects of a 5 or 10 percent mulberry-enriched diet on the blood lipid levels of rats. They found that rats fed mulberry-enriched, high-fat diets (as opposed to mulberry-enriched, "normal" diets) experienced significant decreases in triglyceride, total cholesterol, and LDL ("bad") cholesterol levels, as well as increases in HDL ("good") cholesterol levels. Researchers also noticed that the antioxidant activity in their blood and livers increased, and they attributed these findings to the combination of nutrients in mulberries, including dietary fiber, flavonoids, vitamins, and other compounds.

Indeed, mulberries contain numerous vitamins and minerals, including vitamin C, calcium, magnesium, and iron. The most predominant mineral in mulberries appears to be potassium, a nutrient that is essential for maintaining normal electrical activity of the heart. One cup (125 g) of fresh mulberries boasts around 270 milligrams of potassium, more than the amount in half of a banana. And a single ounce (28 g) of dried mulberries—just a small handful—meets nearly 10 percent of your daily calcium needs.

Inflammation-Reducing Berry with Cancer-Fighting Potential

The heart-protecting anthocyanins in mulberries also help reduce inflammation and boost antioxidant activity in organs like the liver and brain. Animal studies have shown that mulberry extracts can improve memory and learning, and researchers believe that the protective antioxidants in mulberries—like those in blueberries—may help prevent age-related diseases of the brain, including Alzheimer's and Parkinson's disease.

Mulberries also appear to have some cancer-fighting activity, and cell studies have found that their extracts can trigger cell death in certain cancerous cells like glioma cells, which are commonly found in the brain. They may also inhibit the spreading of some cancer cells like those of the skin. Researchers attribute much of their anticancer activity to their rich content of anthocyanins, though it is likely that numerous beneficial antioxidants and phytochemicals are involved.

PUTTING IT INTO PRACTICE

Fresh mulberries are typically harvested in the late spring. These plump, juicy, and sweet berries make great additions to smoothies and salads and can be incorporated into most baked goods or used to make jams and sauces. When fresh mulberries are not in season, dried mulberries are a convenient option, and you can find these sweet and chewy berries in most supermarkets and health food stores. Enjoy them alone as a snack or add to cereals, granolas, and homemade trail mixes. The dried berries can also be used in baked goods and desserts in place of other dried fruits, for an antioxidant boost.

MULBERRY CHEWS

"Dense," "sweet," and "chewy" are three words that best describe these nutritious energy bites. The combination of naturally sweet mulberries and dates along with protein-rich hemp seeds make them a perfect go-to snack. Bring them on long walks, hikes, or bike rides for a natural energy boost.

1 cup (120 g) dried mulberries

1 cup (about 10 to 12, or 178 g) pitted dates

4 tablespoons (30 g) hemp seeds, divided

1 teaspoon lemon zest

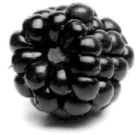

Yield: 12 to 15 chews

Put the mulberries in a food processor and process into a coarse meal. Add the dates and process until a slightly sticky mixture forms. If the mixture appears too dry, add one to two more dates and process. If the mixture is too sticky, add a tablespoon (8 g) of mulberries and process. Transfer the mixture to a medium-size bowl. Add lemon zest and 2 tablespoons (15 g) of the hemp seeds and mix until well combined and evenly distributed (you may need to use your hands). Roll into tablespoon-size (15 g) balls and dredge in the remaining hemp seeds to coat. Store at room temperature for up to 3 days, refrigerate for up to 1 week, or freeze for long-term storage.

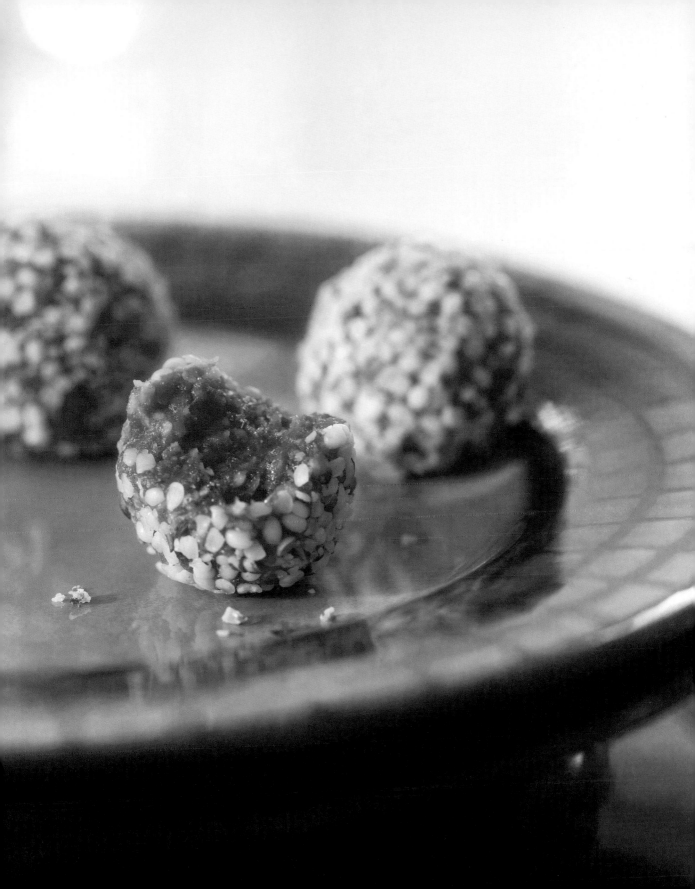

SEA BUCKTHORN BERRY
Nature's Multivitamin

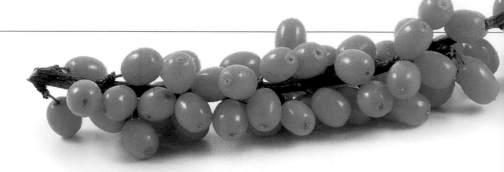

DID YOU KNOW?

Vitamin C–rich foods like sea buckthorn and camu camu berries may help you burn more fat when you work out. Vitamin C helps synthesize carnitine, a compound that turns fat into energy, and getting enough vitamin C in your diet may help you burn more body fat when you exercise. That's right, burn more fat. In a study published in 2006, researchers at Arizona State University found that subjects with marginal vitamin C status burned 25 percent less fat per kilogram (2¼ pounds) of body weight during a sixty-minute treadmill walk than did those with adequate vitamin C status. And those who burned less fat during exercise also became more fatigued—and you know when you get tired, you will stop exercising. So eat vitamin C–rich foods—like berries, peppers, and citrus fruits—every day to support your workouts and your weight.

Sea buckthorn berries are the antioxidant-rich, anti-inflammatory, and immune-boosting berries of a small, thorny deciduous shrub (*Hippophae rhamnoides*) that grows throughout Europe and Asia. These tart, yellow-orange berries were originally harvested in the Himalayas and have been used for centuries as food and medicine to treat conditions ranging from slow digestion and ulcers to skin diseases and soft tissue injuries. Today, these berries are being studied for their potentially beneficial role in the treatment of cancer, heart and liver diseases, and obesity and their healing effects on the skin and digestive tract. Indeed, sea buckthorn berries are reported to have more than 190 active compounds that play a protective role in the body—inside and out—making them a superfood for optimal health.

Nutrient-Rich Super Fruit for Health and Healing

Sea buckthorn berries have been called "nature's multivitamin." They are high in B-complex vitamins and vitamins A, C, E, and K. In fact, they are thought to be one of the most concentrated sources of vitamin C, an antioxidant that helps boost the immune system, speed wound healing, and promote the growth and repair of body tissues. Researchers have found that fresh berries can contain more than 100 milligrams of vitamin C per ounce (28 g), meaning that a small handful will meet around 110 to 130 percent of your daily needs.

Sea buckthorn berries are a good source of minerals like potassium, calcium, magnesium, and iron and boast a pretty unique fatty acid profile. About 70 percent of the fat in sea buckthorn berries is in the form of heart-healthy essential fats, including the omega-6 linoleic acid and the omega-3 alpha-linolenic acid. They also contain smaller amounts of palmitoleic acid (sometimes referred to as an omega-7 fatty acid), a mono-unsaturated fat that has antimicrobial properties and promotes healthy skin and wound healing. In fact, researchers have found that because these berries are rich in beneficial fatty acids, consuming them may help heal damage along the intestinal tract and

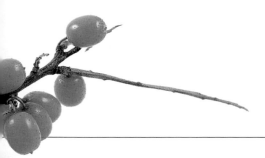

prevent constipation and ulcers. Used topically, oils from sea buckthorn berries and seeds help boost antioxidants in the skin and reduce pain and inflammation caused by burns (including sunburn), eczema, acne, atopic dermatitis, and other skin conditions. And because they are high in vitamin C, they may also help prevent wrinkles and boost the production of collagen.

Clot-Busting, Cancer-Fighting Super Berry

Although some research has shown that vitamin C contributes to about 75 percent of the antioxidant activity in sea buckthorn juice, these berries are also loaded with heart-healthy, cancer-fighting phytochemicals, including flavonoids like quercetin and carotenoids like beta-carotene. Researchers have found that these phytochemical-rich super berries and their juices can trigger cancer cells to self-destruct, inhibiting the growth and proliferation of leukemia and colon, prostate, stomach, and skin cancers. And these same cancer-fighting compounds are also good for the heart.

The flavonoids in sea buckthorn berries help prevent blood clots that may increase your risk of heart attack and stroke. And the berry's seeds are rich in a cholesterol-lowering compound called beta-sitosterol, which may also help regulate blood pressure and lower blood sugar and triglyceride levels—important factors in heart disease and diabetes.

PUTTING IT INTO PRACTICE

Sea buckthorn berries and their juice are quite tart. Although you can purchase sea buckthorn berry juice in a blend of sweeter juices, which often include apple, pineapple, or grape, I recommend buying pure, 100 percent sea buckthorn berry juice. Although it is tart, you can add a small amount—about 2 ounces (¼ cup [60 ml])—to your own freshly pressed juices or blended smoothies. And those 2 ounces of juice will deliver almost 40 milligrams of vitamin C—45 to 55 percent of your daily needs—without the excess sugar from bottled juice blends.

SEA BUCKTHORN BERRY SMOOTHIE

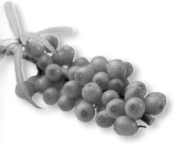

This smoothie combines the sweet flavors of pineapple and mango with the tartness of the sea buckthorn berry. Pineapple is rich in bromelain, an enzyme known for its inflammation-reducing properties, and mango is rich in immune-boosting antioxidant vitamins A and C. When combined with sea buckthorn berry, these power fruits create a superfood smoothie for health and healing.

1½ cups (355 ml) filtered water
¼ cup (60 ml) sea buckthorn berry juice
1 cup (165 g) frozen pineapple chunks
1 cup (175 g) frozen mango chunks
½ teaspoon pure vanilla extract
½ vanilla bean, scraped, or additional ½ teaspoon pure vanilla extract

Combine all the ingredients in a high-speed blender and blend until smooth.

Yield: 2 servings

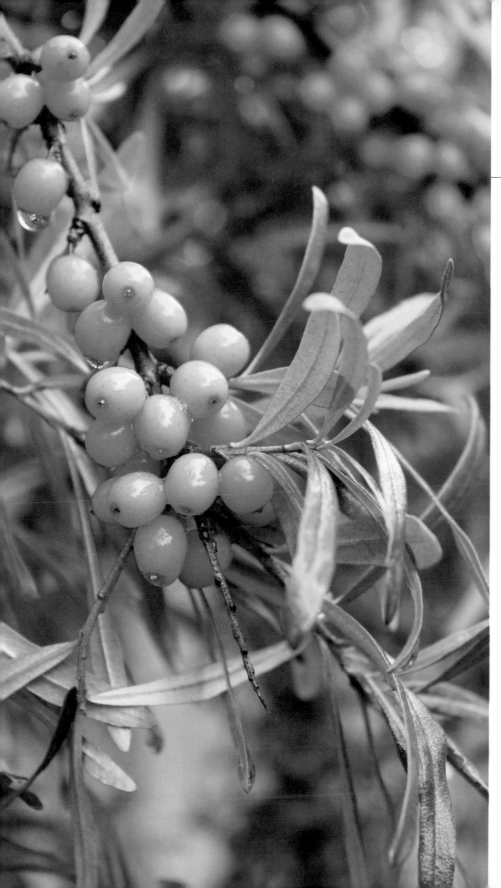

SUPERFOOD KITCHEN TIP: CHOOSING BOTTLED JUICES

I recommend choosing fresh fruits and vegetables—with their beneficial fiber, protein, and enzymes—over bottled juices. However, several of the superfoods in this book (for example, sea buckthorn berries, mangosteen, and noni) are most commonly sold as bottled juices. Here are a few guidelines for choosing bottled juices:

1. Choose only 100 percent, pure juice.

2. Add a small amount—1 to 2 ounces (28 to 60 ml) of a juice concentrate (that you dilute with water) or 2 to 4 ounces (60 to 120 ml) of juice *from* concentrate (meaning it has already been mixed with water)—to sparkling water or your own freshly pressed juices or blended smoothies.

3. Avoid juice blends and products with added sugar or artificial sweeteners, preservatives, colorings, or flavorings—even added vitamins, minerals, and herbs. You want to soak up the benefits of the synergistic blend of naturally occurring nutrients in whole superfoods and their juices.

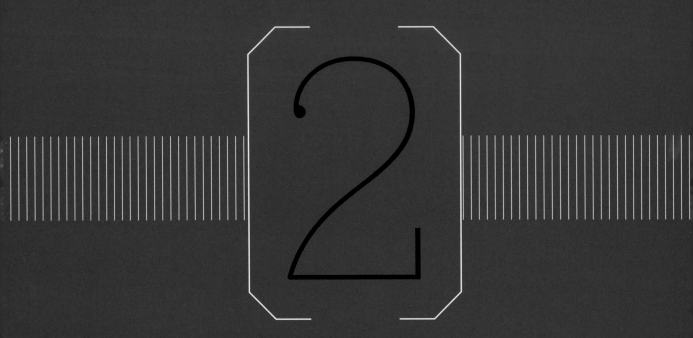

SUPER FRUITS

*Avocado, Cacao, Cherry, Coconut,
Cupuaçu, Mangosteen, Grapes, Noni,
Olive, Pomegranate*

The super fruits on this list include a diverse mix of power foods for optimal health and beauty. From boosting your mood and metabolism to protecting the heart and fighting cancer, these foods are packed with high levels of free radical–scavenging antioxidants and health-promoting phytonutrients. And a few of these super fruits, such as avocados, cacao, coconut, and olives, are rich in beneficial fatty acids that are good for your heart, skin, and even your waistline.

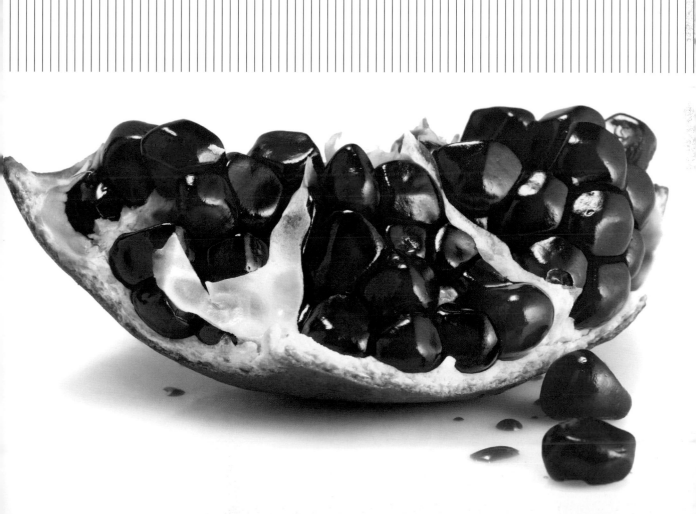

AVOCADO
Heart-Healthy Super Fruit

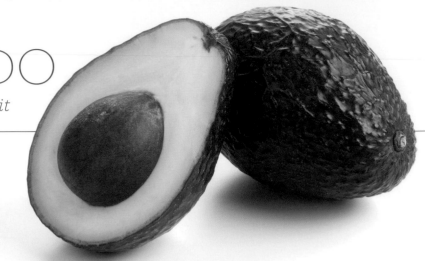

SPOTLIGHT: LUTEIN

Lutein is one of more than six hundred types of carotenoids, pigments that give fruits and vegetables their rich red, orange, and yellow colors and serve as powerful antioxidants that protect against heart disease and cancer. Lutein protects your eyes from age-related conditions that can lead to vision loss and blindness, such as macular degeneration and cataracts. Avocados have one of the highest lutein levels of any fruit; other good sources include broccoli, corn, and leafy green vegetables like kale, collards, and spinach.

Avocados were once shunned because of their high-fat content and the mistaken fear that they—along with other fatty foods like olives and nuts—would clog our arteries and pack on the pounds. Fortunately, times have changed. We are beginning to look at food for its healing properties, not its caloric and fat content. And we now know that not all dietary fats are created equal; in fact, the beneficial fats in plant foods are necessary for good health. As a result, superfoods like the fat-rich avocado are making their way back onto our plates, and our bodies are thanking us.

Plenty of Potassium Plus Fantastic Fats and Fiber

Avocados are incredibly nutrient-dense fruits that contain nearly twenty different vitamins and minerals. They have almost double the amount of potassium than that of a medium-size banana and are packed with folic acid, magnesium, and antioxidants like vitamin E. They are also an excellent source of dietary fiber, which is good for the gut, heart, and weight. At around 10 grams per cup (146 g), they easily meet about a third your daily fiber needs. But what really elevates avocados to superfood status is their abundance of heart-healthy fats and a diverse mix of cancer-fighting carotenoids.

Chock-Full of Cancer-Fighting Carotenoids

It's no secret that avocados are rich in fat, given their creamy, buttery texture. Fortunately, more than half of that fat is in the form of heart-healthy monounsaturated fatty acids like oleic acid. Diets containing these fats may actually help improve cholesterol and triglyceride levels and lower the risk of heart disease. In a study published back in 1996, researchers looked at the effects of avocados on subjects with mildly elevated cholesterol levels. They found that an avocado-enriched diet lowered total cholesterol, LDL ("bad") cholesterol, and triglyceride levels while raising HDL ("good") cholesterol levels. So incorporating healthy fats into your diet—rather than avoiding fat altogether—is a simple step toward heart health.

Avocados are also full of carotenoids, powerful antioxidants that protect against cancer and heart disease. In a 2011 study, researchers at Ohio State University found that avocados prevented the growth and proliferation of both precancerous and malignant oral cancer cells, and a 2005 study conducted at the University of California found that extracts of avocado inhibited the growth of prostate cancer cells. Researchers believe that the combination of phytochemicals in avocados—including various carotenoids—may be responsible for its cancer-fighting effects.

PUTTING IT INTO PRACTICE

Avocados are available year-round in nearly every supermarket, though their peak season is typically from March through August. Their nutrient content varies according to variety, climate, and how they are cultivated. The most popular variety in the United States is the California-grown Haas avocado, which appears to have higher concentrations of heart-healthy fats and other nutrients than varieties grown in Florida.

When choosing avocados, I recommend buying unripe fruits and allowing them to ripen on your countertop. Unripe avocados will feel firm to the touch, whereas ripe avocados will yield to gentle pressure. Once ripe, avocados can be stored whole in the refrigerator to prevent further ripening (unripe avocados will not ripen if refrigerated).

Avocados can be prepared by slicing lengthwise down to the pit, separating into two halves, and scooping out the pit and flesh with a spoon. Alternatively, you can pierce the pit with a knife to extract it and then peel and slice the avocado.

Like most superfoods, avocados are quite simple to incorporate into your diet. Adding a quarter to half of an avocado to your favorite dish is a great way to boost your intake of healthful fats, increase satiety, and improve the absorption of fat-soluble nutrients and phytochemicals. You can chop and add avocados to bean soups or green salads; mash the flesh to create your own vegetable dip or spread (just mix in a little fresh lime or lemon juice to keep it from browning); or blend into your favorite smoothie or salad dressing for extra creaminess.

TOMATO, CUCUMBER, AND AVOCADO SALAD

SUPERFOOD KITCHEN TIP: SCOOPING AVOCADOS

When scooping the flesh out of an avocado, run your spoon all the way down to and along the skin. The greatest concentration of carotenoids is found in the darker green portion of the avocado, which is closest to the peel.

I grew up on tomato, cucumber, and basil salads made with vegetables and herbs picked straight from our family garden. In this recipe, these garden favorites are combined with creamy bites of heart-healthy avocado.

6	Roma tomatoes, halved lengthwise and sliced thinly
1	medium-size cucumber, peeled, halved lengthwise, and sliced thinly
1	avocado, peeled, pitted, and chopped
½	small red onion, sliced thinly
4	basil leaves, torn
2 to 3	tablespoons (30 to 45 ml) extra-virgin olive oil
1	tablespoon (15 ml) apple cider vinegar
	Sea salt and freshly ground pepper to taste

Combine the tomatoes, cucumber, avocado, red onion, and basil in a serving bowl. Drizzle with the olive oil and vinegar and sprinkle with salt and pepper. Toss to combine. Let stand for 15 to 20 minutes before serving.

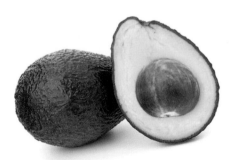

Yield: 4 servings

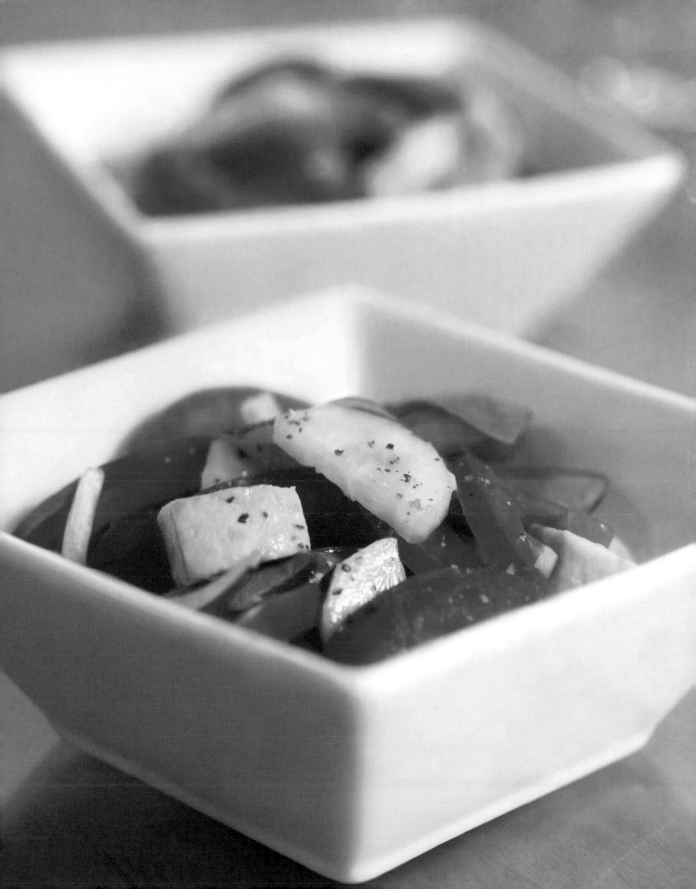

CACAO
Superfood for the Heart and Soul

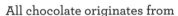

All chocolate comes from the cacao bean, but not all chocolate is created equal. Cacao beans often undergo processing like fermenting, drying, roasting, and alkalizing, which weakens their bitter taste and causes antioxidant losses. Many chocolate products also contain added fat, sugar, emulsifying agents, flavors, colors, preservatives, and milk solids, the latter of which are thought to decrease the absorption of chocolate's beneficial antioxidants. The end result is often a processed chocolate junk food. So skip the highly processed milk chocolate and white chocolate (which contains no chocolate at all) and choose dark and raw chocolate. Your body will thank you.

All chocolate originates from cacao (cocoa) beans, the seeds of football-shaped fruits that grow on the cacao tree (*Theobroma cacao*). Often referred to as "food of the gods," cacao is a beloved superfood with a long history of use in the Mayan and Aztec cultures. Cacao trees are native to Central and South America, where they produce numerous fruits throughout the year, and each fruit contains thirty-five to fifty seeds, which are the cacao beans from which all chocolate is made. Chocolate lovers rejoice: the cacao bean—chocolate in its purest form—has numerous heart-healthy and potentially mood-boosting compounds, making it a superfood for the heart and soul.

Super-Healthy Fats and Flavonoids

Chocolate is a good-for-your body plant food. Two tablespoons (12 g) of raw cacao powder or unsweetened cocoa powder—the amount you might use in a smoothie or cup of hot chocolate—contain about 2 grams of protein and nearly 4 grams of dietary fiber. Cacao is also a good source of minerals that include potassium, magnesium, iron, and calcium.

Although chocolate contains fat—about 12 grams per ounce (28 g) of dark chocolate—more than a third of that fat is in the form of heart-healthy oleic acid, the same monounsaturated fat found in avocados and olives. The remaining fat is saturated, but more than half of it is stearic acid, which, unlike other saturated fats, appears to have no effect on cholesterol levels.

Stress Buster and Mood Booster

Researchers have found that consuming small amounts of chocolate—an ounce (28 g) a few times a week—may help reduce blood pressure, lower total and LDL ("bad") cholesterol levels, increase blood flow to the heart, and make platelets less sticky (and less likely to cause the clots associated with heart attack and stroke).

Chocolate may also help improve blood sugar levels and insulin sensitivity, both of which play important roles in diabetes.

There is some evidence that chocolate may also help boost mood and improve cognition—likely due to its flavonoids and stimulants like caffeine and theobromine. One study found that chocolate helped lessen the symptoms of chronic fatigue syndrome, while another found that consuming a small amount of dark chocolate—just an ounce (28 g) or two a day for two weeks—lowered levels of stress hormones like cortisol (and elevated levels of cortisol may increase abdominal fat and risk of heart disease).

PUTTING IT INTO PRACTICE

When it comes to choosing a healthful chocolate treat, your best choices are high-quality, minimally processed chocolate, including raw chocolate, dark chocolate, and unsweetened, unalkalized cocoa powder. Raw chocolate includes whole cacao beans, cacao nibs (crushed beans), and cacao powders (finely milled beans) that are fermented and slow-dried at low temperatures, but not roasted or alkalized. Beans, nibs, and powders can be tossed into smoothies or used to create raw desserts. Nibs are also a great addition to homemade trail mixes that include a variety of nuts, seeds, and dried berries.

When it comes to choosing chocolate, look for products labeled at least 70 percent cacao (or cocoa) because they have more antioxidants and less sugar than do varieties with a lower percentage of cocoa. A square or two of dark chocolate makes a convenient sweet treat that can be enjoyed a few times a week, or whenever a craving pops up.

Unsweetened cocoa powder is also a good choice but choose powders that are not Dutch processed, as alkalizing contributes further to nutrient losses. You can use cocoa powder in baking or to make your own homemade hot chocolate; simply add a scoop or two to your favorite nondairy milk and sweeten naturally with a little agave or maple syrup. You can also spice up your hot chocolate with inflammation-fighting spices like cinnamon, cayenne, nutmeg, or cloves.

CHOCOLATE FREEZER FUDGE

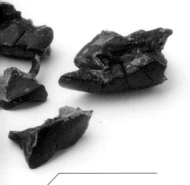

My mom's original fudge recipe was the inspiration for this raw "freezer" fudge. This sweet treat is made from a rich and creamy base of blended cashews, antioxidant-rich cacao powder, slimming coconut oil, and pure, mineral-rich maple syrup—with the added crunch of raw cacao nibs. Enjoy a square (or two) of this decadent snack any time you are craving something sweet and chocolaty.

1 cup raw cashews (140 g), soaked for 1 to 2 hours

½ cup (45 g) raw cacao powder

⅓ cup (107 g) pure maple syrup

¼ cup (56 g) coconut oil

1 teaspoon pure vanilla extract

Pinch of sea salt

¼ cup (32 g) plus 2 teaspoons raw cacao nibs, divided

Drain and rinse the cashews. Place the cashews, cacao powder, maple syrup, coconut oil, vanilla, and salt in a food processor and pulse until smooth and creamy, stopping as needed to scrape down the sides. Transfer the mixture to a medium-size bowl and stir in ¼ cup (32 g) of the cacao nibs until well combined and evenly distributed.

Pour the mixture into a waxed paper–lined 7 × 5-inch (18 × 13 cm) baking dish. Cut the waxed paper to fit the bottom of the pan and rise up and over the two short edges of the dish (this will allow for greater ease at removing the fudge once frozen). Spread the mixture evenly to about ½-inch (1.3 cm) thickness and sprinkle the remaining 2 teaspoons of cacao nibs on top. Freeze until solid, 3 to 4 hours.

Remove from the freezer and lift frozen fudge out of the dish, using the waxed paper. Remove the waxed paper and cut the fudge into twenty-four 1-inch (2.5 cm) squares. Keep frozen.

Yield: 24 squares

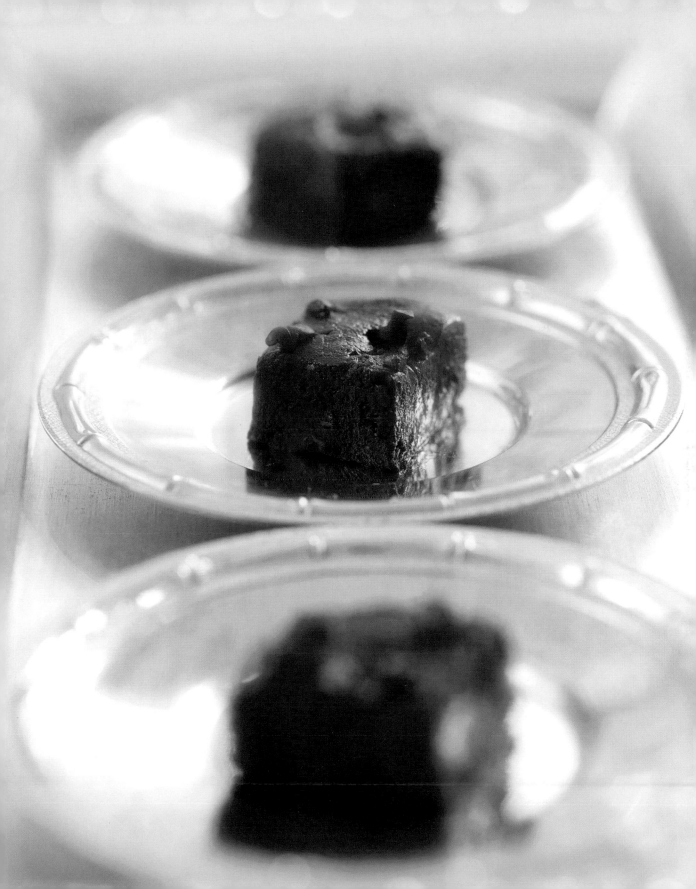

CHERRY

Inflammation-Fighting Super Fruit

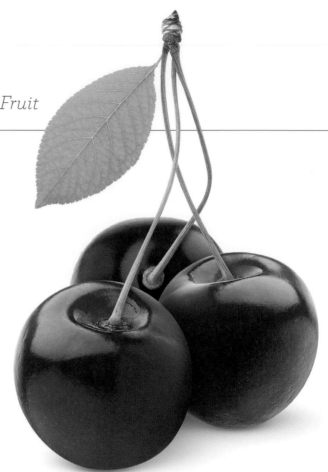

DID YOU KNOW?

The darker the cherry, the more beneficial compounds it contains. In a study published in 2011, researchers in Beijing looked at the levels of beneficial polyphenols in ten different species of cherries with varying colors. They found that red cherries had higher levels of polyphenols and greater antioxidant activity than did bi-colored cherries (which typically contain some yellow). So choose dark red cherries for an extra boost of valuable compounds.

Cherries are small, sweet fruits that are classified into two categories: sweet cherries (*Prunus avium*), which include the popular Bing cherry as well as Lambert, Rainier, and Royal Ann; and tart cherries (*Prunus cerasus*), which include the Montgomery and Morello varieties. Native to Europe and western Asia, cherries are cultivated around the world, including the United States, Turkey, and Iran. Although the tart cherry has received much press over the last few years as a powerful anti-inflammatory food and natural sleep aid, both sweet and sour cherries are nutrient-packed, good-for-your-body super fruits.

Cherries Lower Blood Sugar and Ease Arthritis

The compounds in cherries—including carotenoids and flavonoids like anthoycanins and quercetin—have been shown to inhibit the growth and proliferation of cancer cells, improve heart health (they help lower blood cholesterol and triglyceride levels), and help manage diabetes (they help lower blood sugar levels and reduce insulin resistance). And researchers have found that when you consume cherries, their beneficial compounds can actually block the activity of inflammation-promoting enzymes in the body.

In a study published in 2006 in the

Journal of Nutrition, researchers from the University of California, Davis, found that when twenty healthy men and women supplemented their diet with Bing cherries (about forty-five cherries a day) over a twenty-eight-day period, they experienced an 18 to 25 percent decrease in certain markers of inflammation. Indeed, researchers have found that cherries may help alleviate the pain and inflammation associated with conditions like arthritis and gout.

Natural Sleep Aid

Cherries, specifically the tart ones, may also help you get a good night's sleep. Tart cherries contain high levels of melatonin, a hormone that is produced by the brain and found as a naturally occurring substance in certain foods. Melatonin not only has antioxidant activity but also helps regulate sleep and wake cycles—and the melatonin in cherries may help improve both the quantity and quality of your sleep.

In a study published in 2011 in the *European Journal of Nutrition,* researchers examined the effects of tart cherry juice on the sleep patterns of twenty healthy volunteers. Twice a day for seven days, volunteers consumed 30 milliliters (about 1 ounce) of concentrated tart cherry juice diluted in 235 milliliters (8 ounces) of water first thing in the morning and before bed. Researchers found that those who drank the tart cherry

juice slept longer and had a better quality of sleep than did those who consumed a placebo.

PUTTING IT INTO PRACTICE

Cherries are generally in season from May through August, and if you are like me, you eagerly await the arrival of cherry season. Here in upstate New York, I have picked both sweet and sour cherries at one of our local orchards, and I look forward to the few bags I receive through my summer community-supported agriculture (CSA) farm share. When buying fresh cherries, look for fruits that are firm and unblemished with their stems attached. Cherries can be stored in the refrigerator in a covered bowl or plastic bag, where they will last anywhere from a few days to a week. Avoid leaving them on your countertop, especially during the summer months, as they will quickly spoil. Fresh cherries are great for snacking and make nice additions to salads and smoothies.

When fresh cherries aren't in season, look for unsweetened frozen and dried cherries. Frozen cherries can be tossed into smoothies; one of my favorite combinations is homemade almond milk with a cup (156 g) of frozen cherries and a scoop or two of raw cacao powder. Dried cherries are great for year-round snacking and can be added to bowls of warm cereal, homemade trail mixes, or grain-based dishes like rice and quinoa.

When buying cherry juice, look for brands that contain 100 percent cherry juice and avoid products that contain added sugar or a mixture of cheaper juice blends. You can add a small serving of cherry juice—1 to 2 ounces (28 to 60 ml) of concentrated cherry juice or up to 4 ounces (120 ml) of 100 percent cherry juice from concentrate—to sparkling water, freshly pressed juices, or blended smoothies for a boost of inflammation-fighting antioxidants.

CHERRY DATE BARS

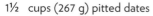

Homemade fruit and nut bars are incredibly simple to make. The natural sugars from fresh and dried fruits combined with healthy fats and protein from nuts and seeds create an ideal snack for at-home or on-the-go enjoyment (and a welcome alternative to a handful of ordinary trail mix). This simple recipe combines high-antioxidant, inflammation-fighting cherries with protein- and calcium-rich almonds. Enjoy these fruit and nut bars at breakfast or snack time.

1½ cups (267 g) pitted dates
1   cup (160 g) dried,
    unsweetened tart cherries
1   cup (145 g) raw almonds

Combine all the ingredients in a food processor and blend until a coarse and slightly sticky dough forms. The dough should stick together when pressed with your fingers. If it feels too sticky, add a tablespoon (9 g) or two of almonds and process. If it is dry or crumbly, add another date or tablespoon (10 g) of dried cherries and process.

Transfer the dough to a waxed paper–lined cutting board, press together into a mound, and flatten with your hands. Cover the dough with waxed paper and use a rolling pin to roll into a ½-inch (1.3 cm) thick rectangle. Trim the edges of the dough to even out, and cut into twelve 1 × 3-inch (2.5 × 7.5 cm) bars.

Yield: 12 bars

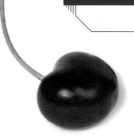

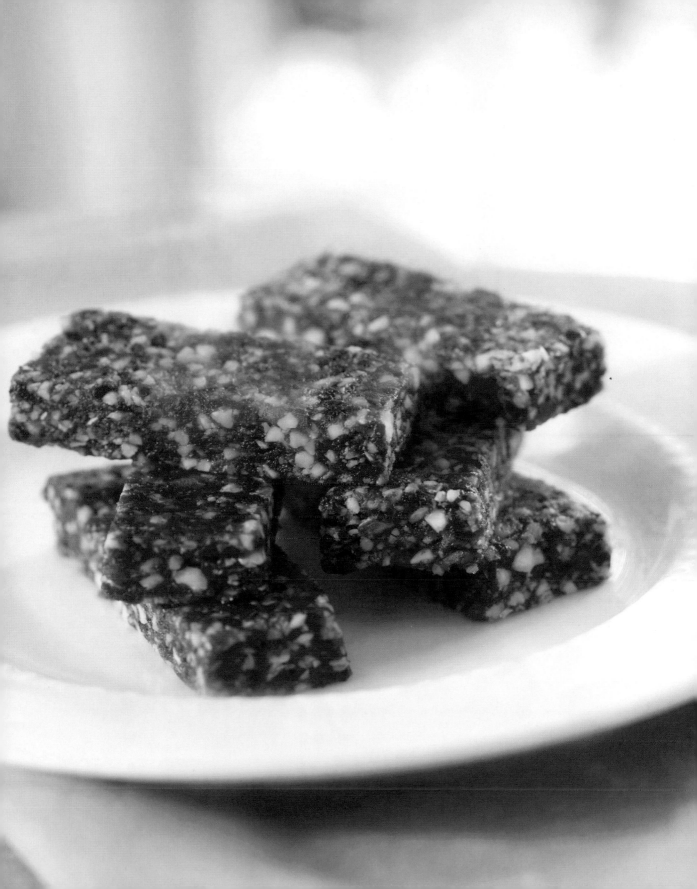

COCONUT
Beautifying Super Fruit

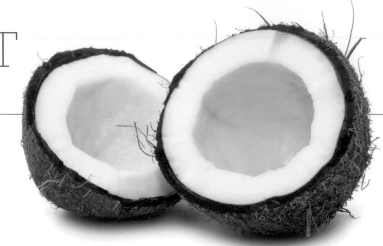

Coconut water is nature's sports drink, rich in potassium (about 600 milligrams per cup [235 ml]) with smaller amounts of sodium (252 milligrams per cup [235 ml]) and energy-producing carbohydrates (about 9 grams per cup [235 ml]). Researchers have found that coconut water is just as effective as traditional sports drinks in maintaining hydration status and promoting recovery between exercise sessions. In addition, coconut water appears to have antioxidant properties that may help neutralize free radicals produced from high-intensity or endurance training. Another bonus: this super drink is free of the artificial colors, flavors, and preservatives found in most commercial sports drinks—chemicals your body can do without!

Coconuts are the fruits of the tropical coconut palm tree (*Cocos nucifera*), and although they are sometimes referred to as nuts or seeds, coconuts are technically classified as drupes, which are fruits with three layers. Coconuts contain a hard outer layer called an exocarp, a fleshy middle layer called a mesocarp, and a woody inner layer known as an endocarp. The coconut you purchase at the market is actually the endocarp (after harvest, the exocarps and mesocarps are trimmed away), which can be cracked open to reveal the edible and highly nutritious coconut meat and water. The beneficial fats in coconut meat and oil may help kickstart your metabolism, keep you slim, heal your gut, fight off bacteria, and help your skin and hair a glow. And coconut water will keep your body incredibly hydrated and energized. In essence, coconut is a superfood that beautifies the body inside and out.

Healthy Fat for a Healthy Weight

Coconuts are high in fat. A tablespoon (14 g) of coconut oil contains about 14 grams of fat and a cup (80 g) of raw coconut meat contains nearly 27 grams of fat—and more than 90 percent of that fat is saturated. However, not all saturated fats are created equal. The saturated fats in coconuts are in the form of medium-chain fatty acids (MCFAs) whose properties and metabolism are very different from the long-chain saturated fats found in animal products. The MCFAs in coconut oil are rapidly and efficiently digested, absorbed, and utilized. They give your body quick energy, boost your metabolism, enhance fat burning, and help prevent fat accumulation in body tissues.

In a 2009 study, researchers looked at the effects of supplementing a reduced-calorie diet with 30 ml (about 2 tablespoons) of either soybean or coconut oil in forty women aged twenty to forty years. After twelve weeks, they found that although both groups lost weight, those on the coconut oil-enriched diet also reduced their waist circumference. Additionally, although those consuming the soybean oil had increases in total cholesterol and LDL ("bad") cholesterol levels, and decreases in HDL ("good") cholesterol levels, the coconut oil group experienced no such effects.

Some studies have found that coconut oil has no effect on cholesterol levels—good or bad—yet others have found that it may help lower cholesterol and blood sugar levels while improving insulin sensitivity.

Coconut Oil Beautifies the Body Inside and Out

Coconut oil is an excellent source of lauric and other fatty acids, which appear to support the immune system and have antiviral, antifungal, and antimicrobial properties. Internally, they work to inactivate a number of pathogenic organisms like *Helicobacter pylori*, stomach bacteria that may cause ulcers, and other harmful intestinal bacteria. And unlike traditional antibiotics that destroy both the good and bad bacteria in the gut, the fatty acids in coconut oil seem to get rid of harmful bacteria while preserving the colonies of beneficial bacteria your body needs for optimal digestion, nutrient absorption, and immune function.

When used topically, lauric acid–rich coconut oil is also a potent natural moisturizer. It may help alleviate skin conditions like atopic dermatitis, psoriasis, eczema, and acne—all of which may result from bacteria, fungi, and viruses. It also appears to have a high attraction to the proteins in hair and can reduce protein loss when applied before or after washing—which means stronger and shinier hair for you. Keep a jar of coconut oil in the bathroom to use on your hair and skin before and after showering.

PUTTING IT INTO PRACTICE

Enjoying the health benefits of coconuts is simple. I recommend buying fresh coconuts; jars of coconut oil; bags of dried, unsweetened, shredded coconut for baking; and containers of coconut milk and water. Fresh coconuts include both young (white with a conical top) and mature (brown and hairy) coconuts, from which you can crack open and drink the fresh water or scoop out the edible flesh. The coconut meat can be eaten raw and blended into smoothies and desserts.

Coconut oil, which is produced by pressing the oil from dried coconut meat, is also widely available. Look for virgin or extra-virgin coconut oils that have not been hydrogenated. They are partially solid at room temperature, but can be easily liquefied by placing the jar in a dehydrator or bowl of warm water and pouring off the liquid. Most individuals can enjoy a tablespoon (14 g) each day, which contains about 14 grams of saturated fat, while still keeping their saturated fat content below the recommended 10 percent of total caloric intake (about 20 grams of saturated fat on a 2,000-calorie diet). You can add coconut oil to smoothies, use in baked goods as a substitute for butter or margarine, or use to sauté vegetables; it is a very stable oil that is ideal for high-heat cooking.

I recommend plain water as your primary source of fluids, but coconut water is an excellent choice for those needing a little extra hydration—especially to replace excess fluid losses from sweating or during and following a bout of intestinal illness.

Finally, coconut milk, made from a blend of grated coconut meat and water, is a nice nondairy milk option that can be used as a base for smoothies, creamy soups, or anywhere you would use regular milk. You can make your own coconut milk or purchase premade varieties, preferably ones that are plain and unsweetened.

VANILLA ALMOND COCONUT COOKIES

These flourless cookies combine almond meal and shredded coconut with coconut oil and a touch of low-glycemic-index agave syrup for a subtly sweet flavor.

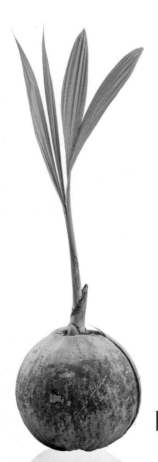

1 cup (112 g) finely ground almond meal

1 cup (80 g) dried, unsweetened, finely shredded coconut

¼ teaspoon sea salt

¼ cup (80 g) agave syrup

¼ cup (56 g) coconut oil

1 vanilla bean, scraped, or 1 teaspoon pure vanilla extract

½ teaspoon almond extract

Preheat the oven to 325°F (170°C, or gas mark 3). Line two cookie sheets with parchment paper.

In a medium-size bowl, stir together the almond meal, shredded coconut, and salt. Set aside. In another bowl, beat together the agave syrup and coconut oil at medium speed using an electric mixer. Beat in the scraped vanilla bean and almond extract. Gradually add the dry mixture to the wet, mixing at low speed until combined.

Place small, rounded scoops—about 2 teaspoons of dough per cookie—onto the prepared baking sheets. Bake for 18 to 20 minutes until the tops just begin to turn a light golden brown (they will still feel soft to the touch).

Remove from the oven and let stand on the cookie sheets for 1 minute. Carefully transfer to cooling racks. The cookies will firm as they cool.

Yield: 20 to 22 cookies

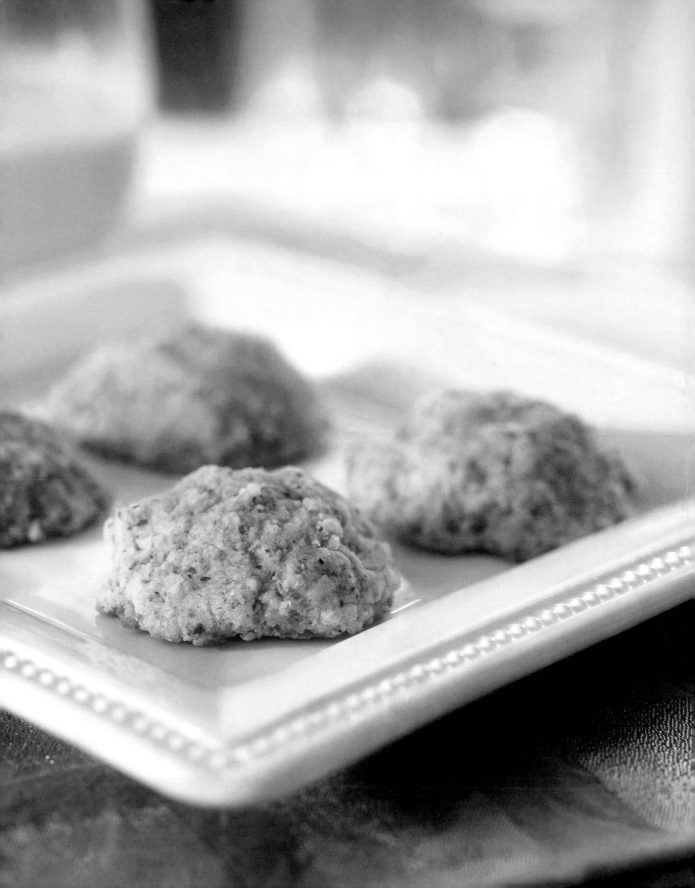

CUPUAÇU
Emerging Super Fruit

<hr />

DID YOU KNOW?

Cupuaçu is one of several fruits of the Amazon that is thought to have great consumer appeal, and in a 2004 study, researchers from Brazil described it as "one of the most popular fruits on the Amazon market" and a food of "nutritional interest." Not only does cupuaçu have a pleasing flavor, which some have described as a unique combination of chocolate, berry, and banana, but it is also packed with valuable phytonutrients, including heart-healthy flavonoids. This combination makes cupuaçu a superfood to watch.

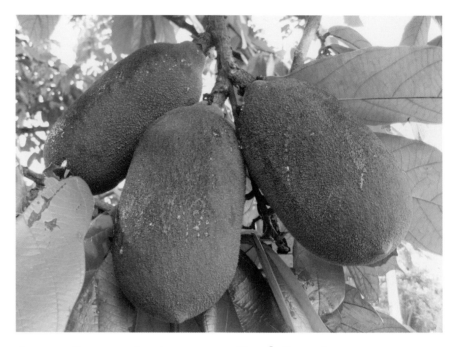

Cupuaçu (koo-poo-ah-su) is a superfood that is just beginning to gain worldwide recognition. Admittedly, I learned of this fruit only a few years back when *The Today Show* did a news piece on five "life-changing" foods that included açai berries, seaweed, and cupuaçu. In that segment, the host of *Bizarre Foods with Andrew Zimmern* described it as a "pharmacy in a fruit" and the "next great superfood." The research is only just beginning to surface on the rich nutrient content and purported health benefits of this tropical fruit whose popularity is slowly but surely growing.

South American Super Staple

Cupuaçu is the fruit of a tree (*Theobroma grandiflorum*) that is related to the cacao tree and native to Brazil. It is cultivated throughout South America and harvested between January and June, with peak abundance occurring between February and April. Although it has been described as one of the most popular fruits in the Amazon, it is only just beginning to be exported worldwide.

Like the coconut, cupuaçu is technically a drupe, which is a fruit with three layers. The endocarp, or inner layer, consists of both a fleshy pulp and seeds, with the flesh mak-

66 | POWERFUL PLANT-BASED SUPERFOODS

ing up about 40 percent of the fruit, and the seeds about 18 percent. The edible pulp is used in the processing of juice, ice cream, candy, jam, and liquors—and is a rich source of health-promoting nutrients.

Rich in the Right Fats

Cupuaçu has a rich combination of proteins, fats, and sugars, along with minerals like zinc and copper, and health-promoting phytochemcials. Although it is about 50 percent sugar, this amount is less than most tropical fruits. It is also packed with more protein than most tropical fruits and boasts about seventeen different amino acids. In addition, cupuaçu contains a variety of fatty acids, and nearly 40 percent of those fats are in the form of heart-healthy and inflammation-reducing oleic and alpha-linolenic acids. Oleic acid is a heart-protective monounsaturated fat also found in açai berries, avocados, and olives, while alpha-linolenic acid (ALA) is the health-promoting omega-3 fatty acid found in chia and flax seeds. ALA helps reduce inflammation, prevent chronic diseases like heart disease and arthritis, and support brain development.

Antioxidants that Beautify the Body

Cupuaçu is high in phytonutrients with strong antioxidant and anti-inflammatory activities. It contains a number of polyphenols, including theograndins, along with at least nine other flavonoids, such as catechin, epicatechin, quercetin, and kaempferol. In cell studies, theograndins, which appear to be somewhat unique to cupuaçu, have demonstrated both strong antioxidant activity and the ability to destroy cancer cells. As a group, flavonoids are among the most abundant antioxidants in the diet, and they have been implicated in everything from lowering the risk of chronic diseases like heart disease and cancer to promoting lung health.

As a result of its high levels of antioxidents and fats, cupuaçu butter is often incorporated into various skin creams. The butter is a luxuriant and creamy emollient that is produced by cold-pressing, refining, and filtering the seeds of the cupuaçu tree. It is commonly added to beauty products to help heal dry and damaged skin, hair, and lips.

PUTTING IT INTO PRACTICE

Cupuaçu is still relatively hard to find outside of South America. You will most likely find cupuaçu in your local health food store or from online retailers that sell it in the form of a juice or powder. Juices and powders can be incorporated into your own freshly pressed juices and blended smoothies. If you purchase the juice, select brands that contain 100 percent, pure cupuaçu juice rather than blended juices or those with added sugars.

CUPUAÇU BANANA SHAKE

Cupuaçu has a sweet taste that is like a cross between chocolate, berries, and bananas. This smooth and creamy shake preserves that sweet flavor by combining it with two simple ingredients: water and frozen bananas.

1½ cups (355 ml) filtered water
2 frozen bananas
¼ cup (22 g) cupuaçu powder

Combine all the ingredients in a high-speed blender and blend until smooth.

Yield: 2 servings

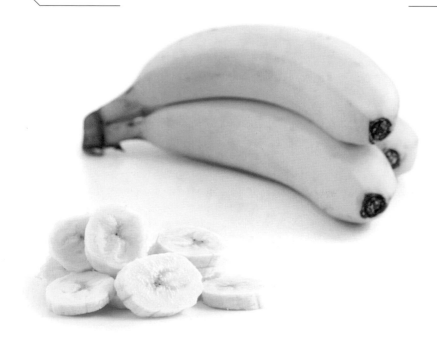

MANGOSTEEN
Queen of Fruit

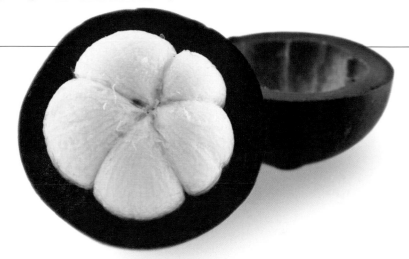

Mangosteen is the tropical fruit of a tree (*Garcinia mangostana*) native to Southeast Asia. Often called the "queen of fruit" in Thailand for its delicious flavor, mangosteen has a long history of use in folk medicine because of its nutritional and medicinal properties. For centuries, traditional healers have used mangosteen to treat abdominal pain, ulcers, and dysentery. Topically, it has been used to treat skin conditions like eczema and infections. And the leaves and bark of the tree have been used to create medicinal drinks. Indeed, researchers are discovering the many potential health benefits of mangosteen—from reducing inflammation and targeting fat cells to fighting cancer and treating acne—making mangosteen a super fruit for super health.

Free Radical–Scavenging, Infection-Fighting Fruit

Mangosteen has been described as an antioxidant-rich, anti-inflammatory, antitumor, antiallergic, antibacterial, and antifungal food. This tropical fruit is high in xanthones, a group of polyphenols that is largely responsible for its antioxidant and anti-inflammatory power. One of the most active xanthones in mangosteen, alpha-mangostin, has a superior ability to scavenge cell-damaging free radicals—comparable to that of the carotenoids in avocados and pumpkins and even greater than the allicin in garlic or melatonin in tart cherries.

The health benefits of mangosteen, including its potent antibacterial and antifungal properties, largely stem from its xanthone content. Mangosteen is well known for its beneficial effects on acne-prone skin, and several recent studies have found that these compounds can reduce inflammation in skin cells and inhibit the growth of acne-causing bacteria. Some research has also found that they can act on certain strains of bacteria (like methicillin-resistant *Staphylococcus aureus*, or MRSA) that are typically not responsive to traditional antibiotic treatments. And in a study published in 2009, researchers found that alpha-mangostin was even more effective in killing *Candida albicans*, a common oral fungus, than were two frequently prescribed medications.

The infection-fighting xanthones in mangosteen also appear to have strong anticancer activities. In a laboratory study published in 2003, researchers found that alpha-mangostin caused the self-destruction of leukemia cells, and within seventy-two hours of treatment, it had completely suppressed their growth. In cell and animal studies, researchers have found that mangosteen-derived xanthones can inhibit the growth and proliferation of a variety of cancer cells, including those of the breast, prostate, lung, and colon. In the case of prostate and breast cancers, researchers have also found that they can prevent metastasis (or spreading) to other organs and glands like the lymph nodes.

Compounds in Mangosteen Target Fat Cells

One growing area of research is the potential role of foods like mangosteen in preventing or treating obesity. Through cell studies, researchers are finding that the polyphenols in plant foods may help break down the stores of fat in cells and stop the production of new fat cells. In a study published in 2012, researchers from Beijing found that alpha-mangostin extracts reduced the activity of an enzyme involved in fat production. As a result, it caused preadipocytes (cells that will develop into fat cells) to self-destruct, reduced the accumulation of fat in mature fat cells, and triggered the breakdown of fat within those cells. Although more research is needed (especially in determining whether what occurs in these cell studies can be duplicated in the body), filling your plate with polyphenol-rich foods like mangosteen, blueberries, green tea, grapes, and citrus fruits, may all prove to help in the battle of the bulge.

PUTTING IT INTO PRACTICE

Mangosteen is a round, mandarin-size fruit with a dark purple shell and inner white edible flesh and seeds. Although the fresh fruits are not commonly found outside of the tropical areas where they are cultivated, mangosteen juices and powders are becoming more widely available at local supermarkets and health food stores. Try adding a splash—about 2 ounces (¼ cup [60 ml])—of 100 percent juice or a scoop of dried powder to your favorite freshly pressed juices or smoothies. Researchers have found that as little as 2 ounces (60 ml) of mangosteen juice are enough to raise antioxidant levels in the body.

MANGOSTEEN
COOLER

This mildly sweet and creamy drink is rich in ingredients that will beautify the body—especially the skin. The antioxidants in mangosteen, collagen-building trace minerals like silica in cucumbers, inflammation-fighting power of ginger and pineapple, and medium-chain fatty acids in coconut oil are a great combination for both skin and fat cells.

1 cup (235 ml) filtered water

¼ cup (60 ml) mangosteen juice

2 medium-size cucumbers, sliced

1½ cups (288 g) frozen pineapple chunks

1 tablespoon (14 g) coconut oil

1 teaspoon grated fresh ginger

Combine all the ingredients in a high-speed blender and blend until smooth.

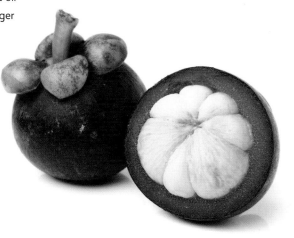

Yield: 2 servings

GRAPES

Heart-Healthy Super Fruit

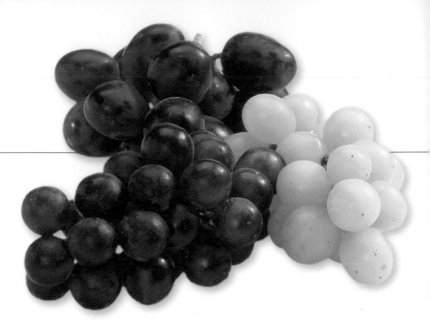

DID YOU KNOW?

A study published in 2007 reported that two-thirds of people who regularly consume supplements take a resveratrol supplement, and unfortunately, there is little research to support its use. A review published in 2011 noted that resveratrol supplements are not likely to offer health benefits in dosages outside of those that can be obtained from the diet, and researchers are not entirely clear about the effects of resveratrol from a pill versus food or the long-term dosing effects of these supplements. As with any superfood, choose real food, not supplements. Resveratrol is found in high concentrations in the skins of red grapes, red wine, grape juice, cranberries, mulberries, and peanuts.

Grapes, from the *Vitis* genus of plants, are a popular fruit in the United States, consumed raw and in juices and wine. According to the California Table Grape Commission, the amount of fresh grapes consumed in this country adds up to about 8 pounds (3.6 kg) of grapes per person per year. That's a lot of grapes and fortunately, a lot of health-promoting compounds we are consuming. Packed with antioxidants and phytochemicals (in levels that rank right up there with blueberries), grapes may reduce your risk of heart disease and cancer and promote a healthy, long life.

Polyphenol-Rich Grapes Are Good for the Heart

Grapes are probably best known for their beneficial effects on the heart—and for good reason. All grapes—green, red, and purple—are high in heart-healthy polyphenols. And eating grapes and drinking the beverages made from them may reduce your risk of heart disease. Researchers have found that the compounds

in grapes help reduce inflammation in the heart, improve blood flow, prevent the clots associated with heart attacks, keep arteries flexible, and lower blood cholesterol and triglyceride levels. That's a lot of heart-healthy action from one small fruit.

When it comes to heart health, researchers are not entirely clear how many servings of grapes or their products you need to consume for benefits. However, some studies have found that you may reduce your risk of heart disease—or the risk factors associated with heart disease (like high blood pressure and cholesterol)—by consuming about 1¼ cups (188 g) of fresh grapes, 1 to 1½ cups (235 to 355 ml) of red grape juice, or a moderate intake of red wine (a maximum of one 5-ounce [150 ml] glass for women or two 5-ounce [150 ml] glasses for men) each day.

Antiaging Benefits of Resveratrol

Grapes may also help age-proof the brain and body. They are rich in resveratrol, probably the most widely known polyphenol in grapes, which helps reduce inflammation and oxidative stress in the body (including areas like the heart and lungs) and may help prevent or treat certain cancers (including those of the colon and breast). This beneficial compound may also help lower blood sugars and improve insulin sensitivity—important factors for those with diabetes. And some studies have found that resveratrol may also help slow the progression of certain age-related diseases.

In animal studies, mice treated with resveratrol tend to have better bone density, reduced cataract formation, improved memory and cognition, and even better balance and motor skills—all conditions associated with aging. And in a study that followed two thousand adults for ten years, researchers found that drinking grape and similar juices more than three times a week reduced the risk of developing Alzheimer's disease by 76 percent compared to drinking it less than once per week.

PUTTING IT INTO PRACTICE

Fresh and frozen grapes can be enjoyed alone as a snack or tossed into fruit and vegetable salads or smoothies. Grapes can be dried into raisins or used to make jams and pie fillings; however, these products tend to contain very little resveratrol and are high in sugar, so enjoy in moderation. Grapeseed oil can also be used to dress salads and vegetables or in high-heat cooking (it has a relatively high smoke point). The oil contains high levels of antioxidants due to its unique content of proanthocyanidins, which are found only in the seeds.

In addition to whole grapes, enjoy moderate amounts of grape juice and red wine. Add 2 to 4 ounces (60 to 120 ml) of 100 percent grape juice to sparkling water, freshly pressed juices, or blended smoothies for a boost of antioxidants. And if you drink wine, women can consume up to one 5-ounce (150 ml) glass per day and men up to two 5-ounce (150 ml) glasses per day to realize the health benefits of grapes. However, greater amounts can actually increase the risk of certain cancers and cause other health problems like heart and liver disease.

RAINBOW CHARD WITH ROASTED SWEET POTATOES AND GRAPES

SUPERFOOD KITCHEN TIP: CHOOSING GRAPES

All grapes have beneficial polyphenols, but seeded red and purple grapes have the highest levels of anthocyanins, their skins have the highest concentrations of resveratrol, and their edible seeds are the only part of the grape to contain beneficial proanthocyanidins compared to seedless green grapes. So enjoy all grapes, but choose red and purple seeded grapes more often for the biggest antioxidant boost.

Chard is an excellent source of immune-boosting vitamins A and C and bone-building vitamin K, which is found in large quantities in all leafy greens. In this recipe, the chard is not cooked, but gently wilted when tossed with roasted sweet potatoes and grapes. If you don't have chard, simply substitute with any leafy green you have on hand. Kale and collard greens are two of my favorites and also work well in this recipe.

3 medium-size sweet potatoes, peeled and cubed (about 2 pounds [910 g])

1 large onion, sliced thickly

¼ cup (60 ml) extra-virgin olive oil
Sea salt and freshly ground pepper, to taste

2 cups (300 g) red grapes

1 large bunch rainbow chard, stemmed and torn into bite-size pieces

Preheat the oven to 400°F (200°C, or gas mark 6). Spread the sweet potatoes and onion onto a 9 × 13-inch (23 × 33 cm) baking dish. Drizzle with the olive oil, sprinkle with salt and pepper, and toss to coat. Roast for 20 to 25 minutes, stirring occasionally. Add the grapes, toss to combine, and roast for an additional 20 to 25 minutes, stirring occasionally, until the sweet potatoes are tender and browned.

Place the chard in a large serving bowl. While still hot from the oven, transfer the roasted potatoes, grapes, and onions to the serving bowl and toss with the chard until it begins to gently wilt. Season with salt and pepper, to taste. Serve warm.

Yield: 6 servings

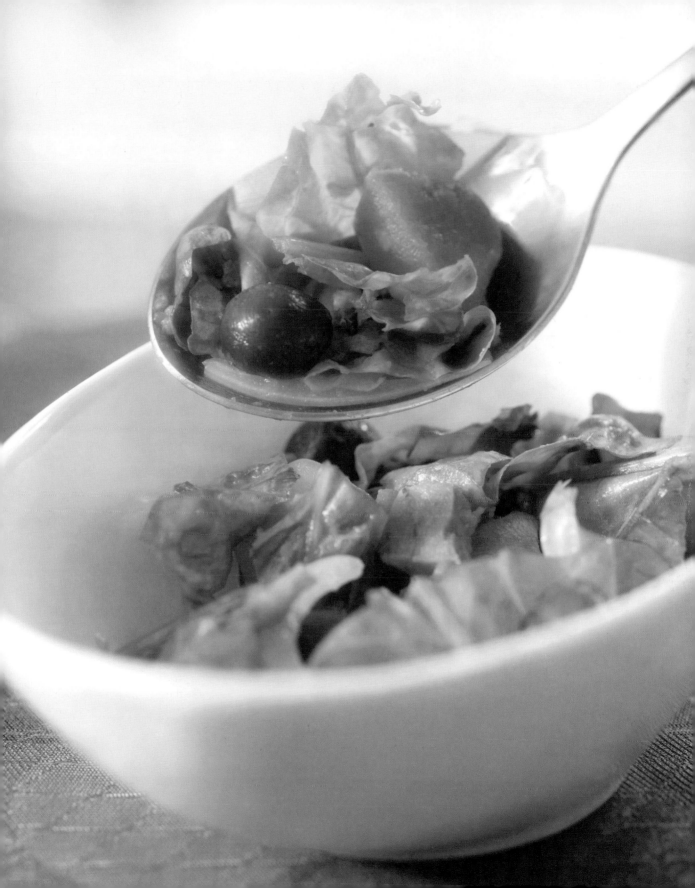

NONI
Polynesian Powerhouse

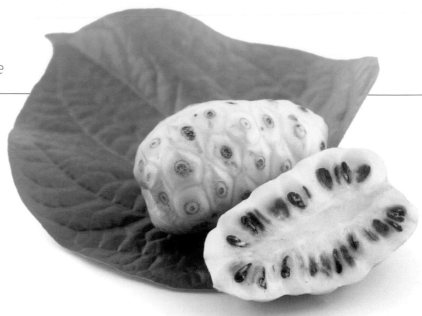

Noni fruits are the yellow, 3- to 4-inch (7.5 to 10 cm), bumpy fruits that grow on small evergreen trees (*Morinda citrifolia*) in Hawaii, Tahiti, and other tropical regions of the Pacific. Although the fruit is enjoyed for its health properties, all parts of the tree—including the leaves and roots—have a long history of use in traditional Polynesian medicine, one that spans more than two thousand years. Described as an antifungal, antibacterial, antitumor, anti-inflammatory, and immune-enhancing plant, noni has historically been used to treat everything from infections and diabetes to arthritis and cancer. And its long history of use combined with a growing body of research is positioning this Polynesian fruit as a modern-day superfood.

Noni May Help Control Blood Sugar

Noni is a good source of magnesium, iron, potassium, and vitamin C. The fruits also contain numerous health-promoting phytochemicals with strong antioxidant and anti-inflammatory properties, including heart-healthy polyphenols, cancer-fighting iridoids, and immune-boosting polysaccharides. Studies have shown that the antioxidants in noni are able to scavenge cell-damaging free radicals and protect body tissues and organs—like the liver and brain—from oxidative damage due to aging or exposure to environmental toxins. In addition, the anti-inflammatory properties of the fruit may help reduce the pain and inflammation associated with conditions like arthritis and gout. And if that weren't enough, some studies suggest that noni may help reduce some of the risk factors associated with heart disease and diabetes.

Indeed, the compounds in noni fruits may help lower total cholesterol, LDL ("bad") cholesterol, and triglyceride levels. And some studies have found that noni may help regulate blood sugar levels by improving insulin sensitivity, stimulating the release of insulin from the pancreas (which helps reduce blood sugars), and delaying gastric emptying (which slows digestion and the release of sugars into the bloodstream). In a study published in 2011, researchers looked at the effects of noni juice and a standard blood sugar-lowering medication on diabetic rats, and they discovered that drinking noni juice had similar effects on blood sugars as taking medication. After twenty days, both the rats that consumed noni juice twice daily and those that received the treatment medication normalized their blood sugars, reducing them by more than 50 percent.

Immune-Boosting Super Fruit

Noni has traditionally been used to fight infections, and this tropical fruit may indeed stimulate the immune system and help fight infections and disease—including cancer.

The compounds in noni, including its beneficial polysaccharides, help activate the immune system's important B and T cells, white blood cells that help your body fight infection. In a cell study published in 2010, researchers found that certain extracts of noni fruit increased immune system activity by up to 35 percent. And these immune-stimulating effects may play an important role

in cancer prevention and treatment because when the immune system is stimulated, it may help suppress the growth of cancerous tumors.

In a study published in 2009, researchers found that the tumors of animals treated with noni (or a combination of noni and an anticancer medication) were 40 to 50 percent smaller than those of the control group. Other studies have found that extracts of noni can destroy small numbers of cancer cells, in some cases by as much as 36 percent—acting, in part, by triggering the self-destruction of those cells.

PUTTING IT INTO PRACTICE

Fresh noni fruits and juices are rarely found outside of the South Pacific, however, bottled juices and dried powders are commonly available in supermarkets and health food stores. Although it is not clear how much noni juice you need to consume to obtain health benefits, two separate University of Illinois studies found that drinking as little as 1 to 4 ounces (28 to 60 ml) of juice daily was associated with improved lipid profiles and a reduced risk of cancer in heavy smokers. As with the juice of any super fruit, I recommend adding a small amount—about 2 ounces ($\frac{1}{4}$ cup, or 60 ml)—of pure noni juice or a few teaspoons of noni powder to freshly pressed juices and blended smoothies for a boost of its beneficial antioxidants. Because noni juice is quite pungent, it blends well with sweeter fruits like berries and bananas.

CREAMY NONI
FRUIT SMOOTHIE

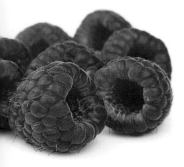

Sweet raspberries and peaches—two late summer power foods—combine with a splash of bitter noni juice in this antioxidant-packed smoothie. The homemade almond milk and banana add a creamy texture—and a boost of minerals like potassium and calcium. Although homemade almond milk is incredibly simple to make, you can substitute with your favorite packaged nondairy milk.

For the Smoothie:

1½   cups (355 ml) Vanilla Almond Milk (recipe follows)
¼   cup (60 ml) noni juice
1   cup (250 g) frozen raspberries
1   cup (250 g) frozen peach slices
1   medium-size banana

Combine all the ingredients in a high-speed blender and blend until smooth.

For the Vanilla Almond Milk:

1   cup (145 g) raw almonds, soaked for 6 to 8 hours
4   cups (950 ml) filtered water
4   pitted dates
1   tablespoon (14 g) coconut oil
1   tablespoon pure vanilla extract
½   vanilla bean, scraped, or additional ½ teaspoon pure vanilla extract

Drain and rinse the almonds. Blend the almonds and water in a high-speed blender for approximately 1 minute. Strain the milk into a separate pitcher using a nut milk bag or strainer. Rinse the blender container with water. Combine the strained milk with the remaining ingredients and blend until smooth. Pour into tightly lidded glass jars and refrigerate. Serve chilled. Shake well before serving.

Yield: 4 cups

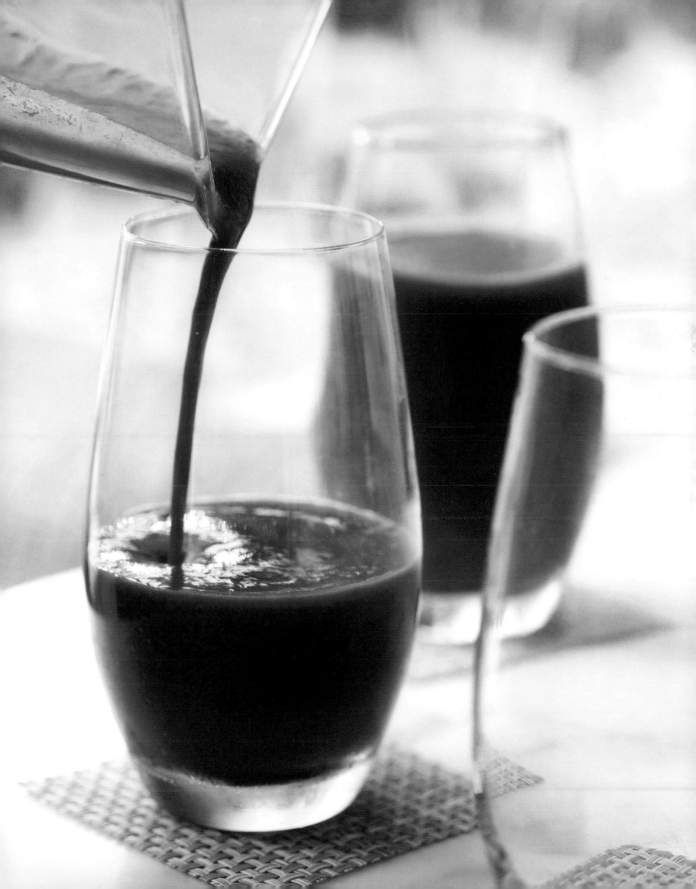

OLIVES

Mediterranean Superstar for the Heart

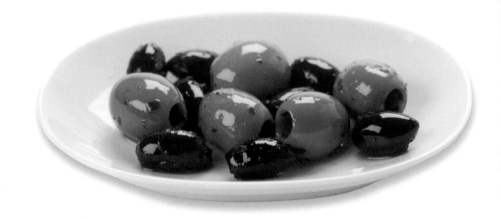

Olives are the small fruits of trees (*Olea europaea*) that grow throughout the Mediterranean. There are an estimated 2,500 different varieties of olives and about 250 of them are cultivated commercially—mostly throughout Spain, Italy, and Greece. Their use in food and medicine goes back more than seven thousand years, and with a rich content of heart-healthy fats and numerous health-promoting phytochemicals, olives are well regarded as a superfood for good health. Their consumption has been associated with reduced risks of both heart disease and cancer, and their potent antioxidant and anti-inflammatory activities may ease arthritis and allergies, while promoting healthy skin.

Healthy Fats and Powerful Polyphenols

Like avocados, olives were once shunned because of their high fat content and the mistaken belief that they would cause weight gain and health problems. A tablespoon (15 ml) of olive oil contains around 14 grams of fat, but more than 70 percent of that fat is in the form of oleic acid, a heart-healthy monounsaturated fat. Researchers have found that eating foods rich in these fats may help lower total and LDL ("bad") cholesterol and increase HDL ("good") cholesterol levels. In fact, early studies found that when people swapped the saturated fat in their diet (commonly found in animal products like butter, lard, cheese, milk, and ice cream) with olive oil, their total and LDL cholesterol levels dropped significantly—by as much as 13 and 19 percent, respectively.

Olives also contain numerous health-promoting compounds, including pigments like chlorophyll and the cancer-fighting and skin-protecting carotenoids like beta-carotene and lutein. These little fruits also contain cholesterol-lowering phytosterols like beta-sitosterol and free radical–scavenging tocopherols. But researchers seem to attribute most of the olive's health-promoting properties to its rich content of polyphenols.

The polyphenols in olives protect red blood cells from injury, prevent LDL cholesterol from being oxidized (which causes plaque buildup and hardening of the arteries), lower blood pressure (olive oil appears to mimic the effects of calcium channel blockers), and prevent the clots that lead to heart attack and stroke. In a study published in 2011 in *Neurology*, researchers found that older adults who regularly consumed olive oil reduced their risk of stroke by 41 percent compared to those who never used it—likely due to the beneficial combination of healthy fats and polyphenols.

Eating Olives May Lower Your Risk of Cancer

Olive oil consumption may reduce your risk of certain cancers, including breast cancer. In a study published in 2006, Italian researchers found that women who consumed more than 30.5 grams (about 2 tablespoons) of olive oil per day were 30 percent less likely to be associated with increased breast cancer risk than those who ate less. The combination of anti-inflammatory fats and

phytochemicals in olives is thought to play a protective role.

Researchers have found that oleic acid may turn off certain breast cancer–promoting genes, and compounds in olives called triterpenes may help stop the growth and proliferation of breast and other cancer cells, including those of the colon, prostate, and skin. Several studies have shown that triterpenes cause cancer cells to self-destruct; in one study, they triggered the self-destruction of more than 80 percent of skin cancer cells.

PUTTING IT INTO PRACTICE

You have likely consumed olives in at least one of their two edible forms: table olives or olive oil. Olives can be green or black, with the only difference being their degree of ripeness (olives will darken as they ripen), and they are often dry-cured or cured in water, brine, or oil to make them less bitter and more flavorful. You can toss olives into salads or pastas, use them in cooking, or create delicious spreads like tapenades. I often enjoy a small serving of plain, marinated, or garlic- or almond-stuffed olives—around five—as a midday snack.

When it comes to olive oil, I recommend using only organic, cold-pressed, extra-virgin olive oil, which is the oil of the first pressing and contains more oleic acid than any other grade of olive oil. Olive oil has a low smoke point and heating it at high temperatures will cause its fats to become unstable—and even form potentially cancer-causing compounds. For that reason, I recommend using olive oil to dress salads, raw or steamed vegetables, and pasta dishes—and for only light sautéing over low heat.

GARLIC ROSEMARY OLIVES

I often use kalamata olives in this recipe, but you can use any combination of oil- and brine-cured olives. They are great for snacking, tossed into salads or pasta, or served alongside other superfoods like seasoned nuts, broken squares of dark chocolate, and seasonal fresh fruits like grapes and strawberries.

3 cups (510 g) kalamata olives, rinsed and drained

3 sprigs fresh rosemary

3 cloves garlic, sliced thickly

¼ cup (60 ml) extra-virgin olive oil

Zest of 1 small lemon

Yield: 3 cups

Combine all the ingredients in a large bowl and mix well. Refrigerate in a tightly lidded container for at least 24 hours, stirring occasionally. Bring to room temperature before serving.

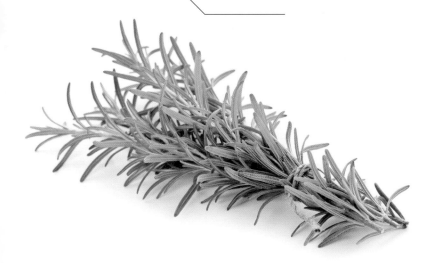

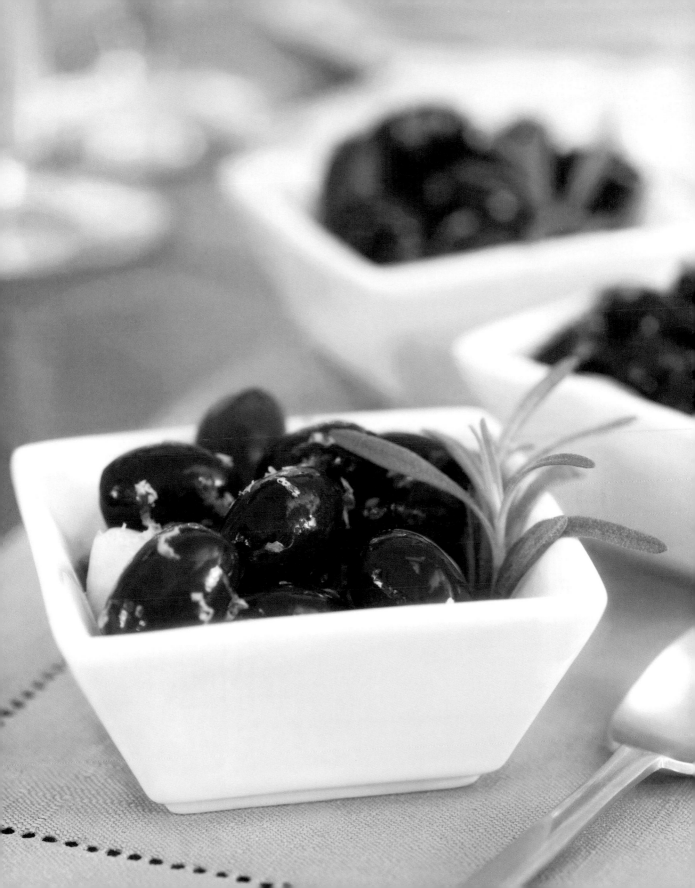

POMEGRANATE

Nature's Power Fruit

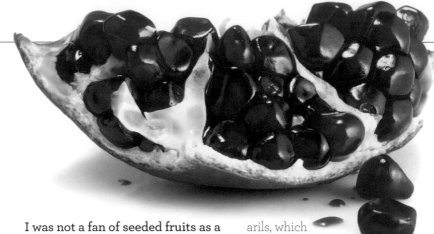

I was not a fan of seeded fruits as a child. And so every fall and winter, I would watch as my grandmother, mother, and older sister dug into the bright red, leathery skins of fresh pomegranates just to get at their clusters of little seeds. They would scoop out the edible seeds and their surrounding juicy, red pulp and eat them by the spoonful. Back then, it seemed like so much work (and mess) for so little reward, but I know better now. The pomegranate (*Punica granatum*), sometimes called "nature's power fruit," is one of the most antioxidant-rich fruits in the world. And consuming the fresh fruits and juices of this superfood provides a delicious way to give your body an antioxidant and anti-inflammatory boost.

Antioxidant-Rich Fruit of the Middle East

Pomegranates are native to the Middle East, but they are cultivated throughout the world, including around the Mediterranean and in the United States. These super fruits are a good source of fiber, vitamin C, and potassium. One cup (174 g) of the arils, which are the seeds and their surrounding juice sacs, boasts an impressive 7 grams of dietary fiber (20 to 30 percent of your daily needs) and more than 400 milligrams of potassium (the same amount as a medium-size banana). Each cup (174 g) also delivers small amounts of fat and protein—nearly 2 and 3 grams, respectively.

But what makes the pomegranate a superstar is its remarkable levels of antioxidants and inflammation-suppressing phytonutrients. Researchers have identified more than 120 different phytochemicals in pomegranates, including rich amounts of heart-healthy and cancer-fighting flavonoids like anthocyanins and tannins like ellagitannins. In a study published in 2008, researchers found that pomegranate juice had the greatest antioxidant capacity of thirteen different juices tested—even more than red wine, green tea, and açai berry juice.

Cancer-Fighting Super Fruit

The combination of flavonoids, tannins, and other phytochemicals in the pomegranate makes it a potent cancer fighter. Researchers have found that extracts of pomegranate and its ellagitannins can inhibit the growth and proliferation of certain cancer cells. Positive effects have been seen in cancers of the breast, lungs, colon, and skin, though the strongest effects appear to be on the prostate.

In a study published in 2006, researchers at the University of California, Los Angeles, tested the effects of pomegranate juice on rising PSA (prostate-specific antigen) levels in men with previous surgeries or radiation due to prostate cancer. (PSA is a test used to detect prostate cancer or other prostate irregularities, and it is also used as a predictor of survival for those with recurrent prostate cancer.) They found that 85 percent of patients who consumed 8 ounces (235 ml) of pomegranate juice daily slowed their rising levels of PSA. In addition, sixteen of the forty-six men in the study actually decreased their PSA levels—four of them by more than 50 percent.

Pomegranates Promote Heart Health

The antioxidants in pomegranates keep the heart and blood vessels healthy. Studies have shown that pomegranate juice may help lower blood pressure, reduce inflammation in the blood vessels, and prevent or reduce the oxidation of LDL ("bad") cholesterol, the latter of which can cause artery-clogging plaques to form. It may also help lower cholesterol levels. In a small-scale study published in 2006, researchers found that subjects with type 2 diabetes who drank 40 milliliters (about 1½ ounces) of concentrated pomegranate juice over eight weeks had significant reductions in both total and LDL cholesterol levels.

PUTTING IT INTO PRACTICE

You can easily incorporate both fresh pomegranates and pomegranate juice into your diet. The fresh fruits offer up beneficial fiber and small amounts of protein and fat that you cannot get in the juice. However, the juices appear to contain more of the beneficial antioxidants than the fruits. The ellagitannins in pomegranates are found in greatest concentrations in the fruit husk, and consuming pomegranate juice—from which the whole fruit, including the husk, is pressed—releases significantly greater amounts of ellagitannins than you would consume by eating the fresh arils alone. However, I recommend enjoying both for good health.

You can eat pomegranate arils alone as a snack or tossed into salads or warm bowls of cereals or grains. Try 100 percent pomegranate juice alone or added to sparkling water, freshly pressed juices, and blended smoothies. Several studies have found that as little as 2 ounces (60 ml) and up to 8 ounces (235 ml) of the juice may have beneficial effects on the heart and markers of heart disease (like high cholesterol and blood pressure).

POMEGRANATE AND WILD RICE PILAF

Wild rice is a naturally gluten-free grain that has slightly more protein than other whole grains (about 8 grams per cup [165 g], cooked) and is a good source of fiber, folate, and minerals like magnesium, phosphorous, and zinc. The combination of wild rice with crunchy, antioxidant-rich pomegranate seeds and chopped apples makes this a hearty and savory autumn dish.

1 cup (160 g) raw wild rice

1 cup (185 g) raw brown rice

4 cups (950 ml) water

1 cup (235 ml) balsamic vinegar

2 cloves garlic, crushed

¼ teaspoon dried thyme

2 teaspoons grapeseed oil

1 medium-size onion, chopped

1 apple, chopped

1 cup (174 g) pomegranate arils

½ cup (73 g) sunflower seeds

Sea salt and freshly ground pepper, to taste

Combine the wild rice, brown rice, and water in large stockpot. Cover and bring to a boil. Reduce the heat and simmer until cooked, about 50 minutes.

In a small saucepan, heat the balsamic vinegar over medium heat and simmer, stirring occasionally, until it becomes syrup-like in consistency and is reduced by half, 20 to 30 minutes. Add the garlic and thyme and simmer for an additional 1 to 2 minutes. Remove from the heat and set aside.

In a large skillet, warm the grapeseed oil over medium heat. Add the onion and apple and sauté until the onion is soft, about 3 minutes. Remove from the heat and set aside.

To assemble the pilaf, place the rice, onions, apples, pomegranate arils, and sunflower seeds in a large bowl. Pour the balsamic reduction over the pilaf and stir to combine. Season with salt and freshly ground pepper to taste. Serve warm.

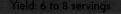
Yield: 6 to 8 servings

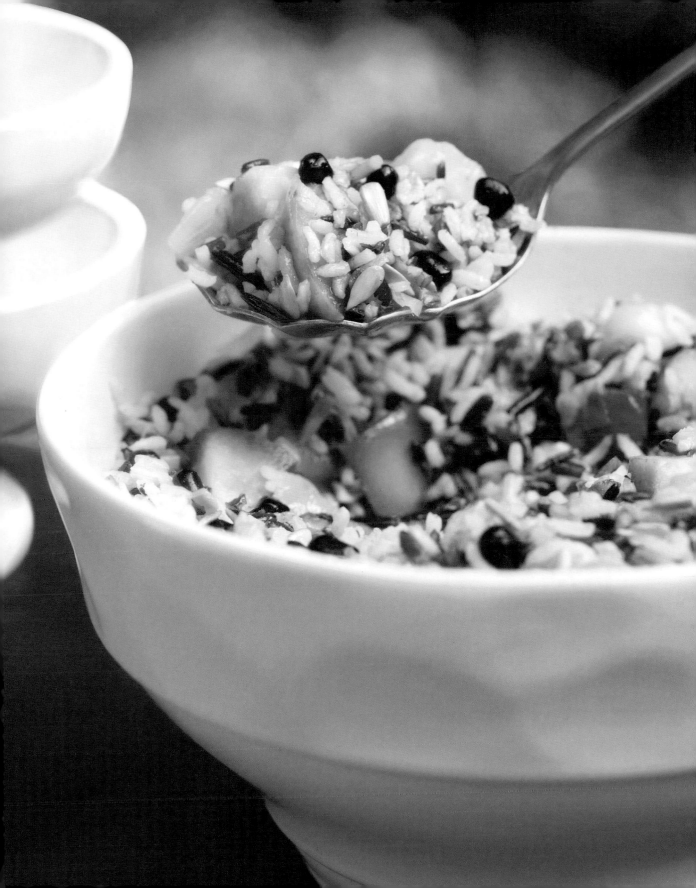

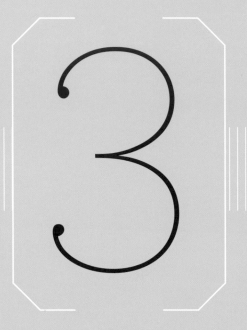

SUPER GREEN FOODS

*AFA Blue-Green Algae, Spirulina,
Broccoli Sprouts, Dandelion Greens,
Kale, Spinach, Chlorella*

Super green foods are packed with blood- and bone-building minerals and vitamins like iron, calcium, and vitamin K; cancer-fighting phytonutrients like carotenoids; and toxin-binding and -eliminating chlorophyll, the pigment responsible for their rich, green color. All greens vary in flavor and nutrition, so enjoy a variety each day to satisfy your taste and nutrient needs. From big raw salads and green smoothies to sautéed greens and soups, it's easy to go green.

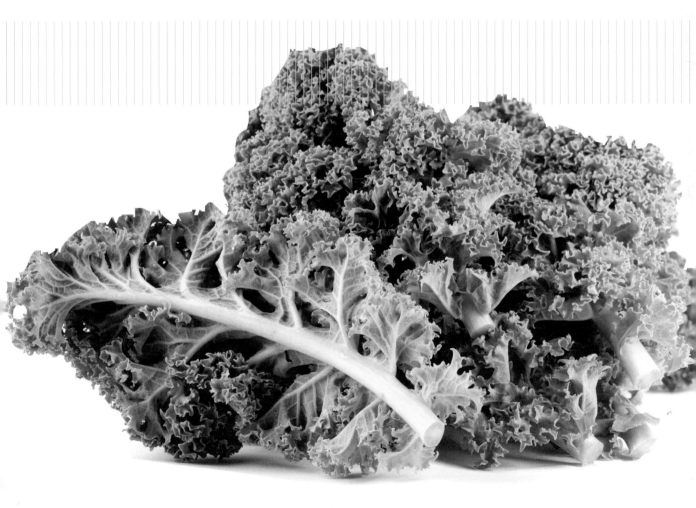

AFA BLUE-GREEN ALGAE
Wild-Harvested Super Algae

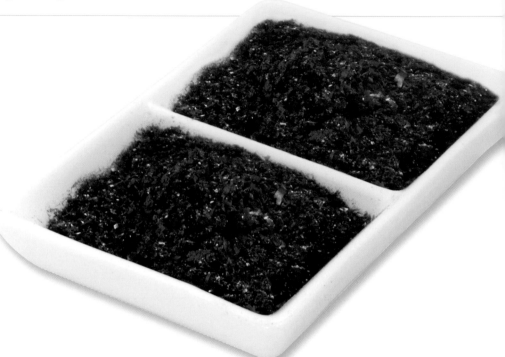

SPOTLIGHT: VITAMIN B$_{12}$

Vitamin B$_{12}$ is an important nutrient for healthy metabolism and nerve function. An estimated 40 percent of the U.S. population—including both vegans and meat-eaters—is deficient in this vitamin, and deficiencies have been associated with fatigue, weakness, anemia, and numbness and tingling in the arms and legs. Despite claims to the contrary, AFA and other plant foods (like unwashed or unpeeled vegetables) aren't adequate sources of vitamin B$_{12}$. Because the only known reliable sources of vitamin B$_{12}$ are animal products, this is one nutrient where supplementing—especially for vegans—is essential.

Aphanizomenon flos-aquae (AFA) are edible blue-green algae that are harvested from Upper Klamath Lake in Oregon. At an elevation of 4,100 feet (1250 meters) above sea level, it has been described as one of the most nutrient-rich lakes in the world. Seventeen rivers feed into it and deposit an estimated 50,000 tons of mineral-abundant silt. Wild-growing AFA have been harvested and processed there for more than twenty-five years. And it is the anti-inflammatory properties and antioxidant power of these unique, edible algae that make them an increasingly popular superfood.

Wild Superfood of the West

AFA contain more than sixty-five different vitamins, minerals, and fatty acids. It comprises all nine essential amino acids as well as tyrosine, a conditional amino acid that is considered essential during times of illness or stress. AFA are also an excellent source of phycocyanin, a pigment responsible for its deep blue-green color and antioxidant power. Also found in spirulina, phycocyanin has been shown to have strong anti-inflammatory properties. In fact, researchers have found that extracts of AFA may help reduce pain and inflammation and have a protective effect on tissues and organs such as the brain, liver, and kidneys.

In addition, AFA may help boost the immune system and promote healing. In a study published in 2010, researchers at the University of South Florida found that certain extracts of AFA may help enhance stem cell production in vitro. And some studies have shown that AFA extracts may aid in activating macrophages and natural killer cells—two special types of cells that help stimulate the immune system while destroying bacteria, viruses, and dead or diseased cells in the body.

Chlorophyll-Rich Superfood May Help Eliminate Toxins

AFA are an excellent source of chlorophyll, a pigment that gives plants their green color and acts as a powerful antioxidant. It is found in all leafy green vegetables, algae like chlorella and spirulina, and green grasses like wheat and barley.

What is exciting about chlorophyll is its potential role in cancer prevention. Researchers have found that chlorophyll attaches to potentially cancer-causing compounds and toxins in the body, preventing their absorption.

In a 2012 study conducted at Oregon State University, researchers tested the effects of chlorophyll on cancer-causing compounds in rainbow trout. In the study, the fish were exposed to moderate levels of a carcinogen and then treated with chlorophyll. The chlorophyll was able to bind with the carcinogen and eliminate it from the body through the digestive tract. The results? Treating the trout with chlorophyll reduced their number of liver tumors by 29 to 64 percent and stomach tumors by 24 to 45 percent.

PUTTING IT INTO PRACTICE

Although AFA are a wild food, you can purchase it frozen or in the form of a powder. Frozen AFA can be thawed and consumed as a liquid alone or diluted with a small amount of fresh juice or water. I recommend adding AFA powder, liquid, or frozen cubes (I often thaw an entire jar of AFA, pour into small ice cube trays, and refreeze) into your own freshly pressed juices or blended smoothies. One major manufacturer recommends starting with a small amount of AFA—about ½ to 1 teaspoon—and increasing intake gradually up to 1 tablespoon (15 ml) or more each day, depending on how your body feels.

Because AFA grow in the same water as other inedible, toxic algae (such as *Microcystis aeruginosa*, which produces a liver toxin called microcystin), there is some concern over accidental contamination that could occur during harvest. For this reason, if you choose to consume AFA, buy only 100 percent pure AFA from a reputable company that can verify that its products have been tested for and found free of contaminants. Also be sure to discuss any supplements you are taking with your health-care provider, especially if you are a woman who is pregnant or breastfeeding. And please, do not attempt to grow or harvest AFA yourself.

LEMONY GREEN JUICE

HOW TO BUILD A BETTER GREEN JUICE

Here are five tips to getting the best nutrition and flavor from green drinks:

1. Prep your produce. Wash fruits and vegetables thoroughly. If you use organic produce, leave them unpeeled unless otherwise specified. I suggest peeling conventional produce to remove additional pesticides. All produce can be left whole or chopped to fit the feed tube of your juicer.

2. Use fresh greens. The longer leafy greens sit in the fridge, the more bitter they taste, so use within a day or two of purchase.

3. Experiment with a variety of greens. All leafy greens have different flavors and nutrient profiles. For example, kale is more bitter but its calcium is better absorbed than spinach. So mix up your greens each day for flavor and nutrition.

4. Add an extra lemon, lime, or apple to your green juice. The citrus flavor will help cut the bitter taste of greens, and adding an apple will make your juice sweeter.

5. Serve cold. Green juices taste better chilled. Refrigerate your ingredients the night before juicing or serve over ice.

This juice is a great introduction to green juices. It is incredibly crisp and refreshing—and lusciously green because of the powerful health-promoting pigments in the leafy greens, green vegetables, herbs, and AFA blue-green algae. If you don't have a juicer, try adding AFA to any of the smoothies in this chapter.

1	head romaine lettuce
3 to 4	stalks kale
3 to 4	stalks celery
1	medium-size cucumber
1	bunch parsley
2	lemons, peeled
1	green apple
1	thumb-size piece fresh ginger, peeled
1	teaspoon to 1 tablespoon (15 ml) liquid AFA

Push all the ingredients except the AFA through a juicer. Add the AFA to the juice pitcher and stir to combine. Serve immediately.

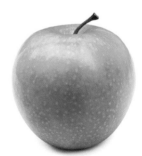

Yield: 2 servings

SPIRULINA
Inflammation-Fighting Super Algae

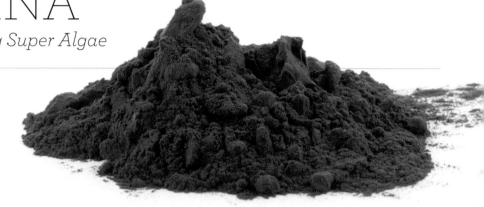

DID YOU KNOW?

Contrary to popular belief, green foods—not orange ones like carrots—help protect your eyes. Leafy greens and microalgae have some of the highest levels of the eye-protecting compounds lutein and zeaxanthin. Some studies have found that diets rich in these two carotenoids can reduce the risk of cataracts by 20 percent and macular degeneration by 40 percent—giving you two more reasons to add more green foods to your diet.

Spirulina is microscopic, freshwater blue-green algae that grow throughout the alkaline waters of Mexico, Asia, central Africa, and the Americas. Consumed for hundreds of years in Mexico and central Africa, spirulina was once harvested from Lake Texcoco (in what is now Mexico City) by the Aztecs, who dried it for use in cakes and broths. Although there are more than a hundred different species of spirulina, three common, edible ones—*Spirulina platensis*, *Spirulina maxima*, and *Spirulina fusiformis*—continue to be explored for their health-promoting potential. From enhancing immunity and easing allergies to lowering cholesterol and removing toxins from the body, researchers are finding that this nutrient- and antioxidant-rich superfood may give your health a super boost.

Protein- and Pigment-Packed Algae

Spirulina is an excellent source of numerous vitamins and minerals, including vitamin E, manganese, iron, and selenium. Sixty to 70 percent of the dry weight of this green food is protein, which includes all nine essential amino acids. Spirulina also contains gamma-linolenic acid, an omega-6 fatty acid that—unlike other omega-6 fatty acids—appears to reduce inflammation, not promote it. The vibrant green color of spirulina is the result of several beneficial plant pigments, like chlorophyll and phycocyanin, which also contribute to its health-promoting properties. Chlorophyll appears to bind to and eliminate potential cancer-causing compounds in the body, preventing their absorption, and phycocyanin may help reduce inflammation while protecting organs like the brain and liver. Spirulina also contains cancer-fighting carotenoids like beta-carotene, though their trademark orange hues are masked by chlorophyll's rich green color.

A Free Radical-Scavenging Antioxidant

The combination of powerful compounds in spirulina—mainly beta-carotene and phycocyanin—contribute to its strong antioxidant activity and ability to protect cells from the damaging effects of free radicals. In 2010, researchers found that spirulina extracts exerted greater free radical–scavenging abilities than did extracts of phycocyanin alone (suggesting that there is a likely synergistic effect between its compounds).

Researchers have also found that the compounds in spirulina may help block pathways in the body that can lead to inflammation. As a result, it may help reduce pain and inflammation associated with arthritis; ease allergy symptoms by blocking the release of histamine, which causes runny nose, itchy eyes, and sneezing; and even boost the growth of beneficial bacteria in the gut (like *Lactobacillus acidophilus*), which may help calm irritable bowel syndrome, improve digestion and nutrient absorption, and treat conditions like diarrhea following antibiotic use. Spirulina may also help boost the immune system by increasing the production of antibodies and other cells that are useful in fighting off infections and even cancer.

Cholesterol-Lowering Super Green

Spirulina may also help reduce some of the risk factors associated with heart disease, such as high cholesterol levels. Several animal studies have found that diets supplemented with spirulina may lower total and LDL ("bad") cholesterol, increase HDL ("good") cholesterol levels, and reduce the accumulation of fat in the liver that often occurs from eating a high-fat, high-cholesterol diet. In a study published in 2010, researchers looked at the effects of a spirulina-enriched, high-cholesterol diet in rabbits with elevated cholesterol levels. After eight weeks, they found that a 1 percent spirulina-enriched diet reduced LDL cholesterol by more than 26 percent, while a 5 percent spirulina-enriched diet lessened LDL cholesterol by more than 40 percent. Researchers also found that both groups had lower total cholesterol levels and increased HDL cholesterol levels.

Similar findings have been seen in human studies. In 2007, researchers looked at the effects of spirulina supplementation on the blood lipids of thirty-six men and women over a six-week period. After consuming 4½ grams (approximately 1 tsp) of spirulina each day, subjects experienced significant decreases in triglyceride, LDL cholesterol, and total cholesterol levels, as well as improvements in blood pressure. In fact, following treatment, the prevalence of both high cholesterol and triglycerides was cut in half. Nearly 28 percent of subjects had elevated cholesterol levels prior to treatment, whereas only 14 percent had elevated lipids after treatment.

PUTTING IT INTO PRACTICE

Spirulina can be found in most supermarkets and health food stores and is typically available as a tablet or dried powder. Powders can be added to freshly pressed juices or blended smoothies, sprinkled into salads, or whisked into homemade salad dressings. Many spirulina-based products are also becoming more available, including raw food bars and cookies. You can also make your own treats, using a mixture of dried fruits, nuts, spirulina, and other superfood powders. This super green is excellent when combined with raw cacao powder, maca powder, and coconut—three additional top superfoods.

CHOCOLATE ALMOND GREEN SHAKE

**SUPERFOOD KITCHEN TIP:
BLENDING AND JUICING**

Both juicing and blending can benefit health. They provide a simple—and delicious—way to get a big boost of vitamins, minerals, live enzymes, and phytonutrients. So what's the difference between the two? Juicing tends to be gentler on the digestive tract because it floods your body with nutrients from the fruits and vegetables you juice—without the fiber. For this reason, juices tend to be more rapidly digested and absorbed, making them ideal as a pre-meal or between-meal snack. By contrast, smoothies provide the nutrients of the fruits and vegetables you blend—plus the fiber. For this reason, they tend to be more slowly digested and absorbed (especially when they include protein-rich nuts, seeds, and powders), making them an ideal meal in a glass. Enjoy both juices and blended drinks for good health!

This rich and creamy smoothie combines the complementary flavors and antioxidant and inflammation-fighting powers of raw cacao, goji berries, and spirulina with a sprinkle of stress-busting maca and generous scoop of protein-, calcium-, and fat-rich almond butter. Enjoy this sweet shake for breakfast—or any time you are craving a more substantial but easy-to-digest meal for sustained energy.

1½ cups (355 ml) filtered water
¼ cup (60 g) raw almond butter
2 medium-size frozen bananas
2 dates
¼ cup (23 g) dried goji berries

2 tablespoons (12g) raw cacao powder
2 teaspoons (10 g) raw maca powder
1 serving-size scoop (per manufacturer) spirulina-containing green powder

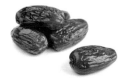

Combine all the ingredients in a high-speed blender and blend until smooth.

Yield: 2 servings

BROCCOLI SPROUTS
Cancer-Fighting Super Sprout

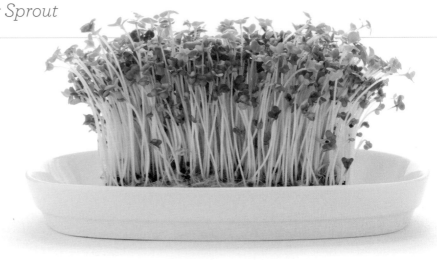

Sulforaphane is a potent cancer-fighting compound that is produced in the body after you consume broccoli and broccoli sprouts. Researchers have found that sulforaphane helps inhibit the growth and spread of certain cancer cells, including those of the breast, prostate, cervix, and bladder. It is also involved in certain detoxification pathways in the body that help prevent toxins you are exposed to from becoming carcinogenic. Good sources of sulforaphane include cruciferous vegetables like cauliflower, cabbage, and Brussels sprouts.

Sprouts are the ultimate live super-foods. These three- to seven-day-old plants are a concentrated source of important vitamins, minerals, enzymes, and phytochemicals. In fact, they have just as much—if not more—of the same nutrients found in mature plants. Another benefit: Sprouts are usually easier to digest and their nutrients are better absorbed than their mature counterparts, in part because of their abundance of live enzymes. From grains and legumes (such as peas and lentils) to radish and broccoli seeds, many foods can be sprouted. And broccoli sprouts—with their impressive levels of cancer-fighting compounds—are a standout among sprouts and a living super-food for the body.

Sprouting More Glucosinolates than Broccoli

Broccoli and broccoli sprouts contain compounds called glucosinolates. When you eat broccoli or its sprouts, these glucosinolates are converted in the body to active cancer-fighting isothiocyanates, more specifically, sulforaphane. Despite both being powerful cancer-fighting foods, broccoli sprouts contain much higher levels of glucosinolates than mature broccoli. Researchers at the Johns Hopkins University School of Medicine found that three-day-old broccoli sprouts contain up to fifty times higher levels of glucoraphanin (a glucosinolate in broccoli) than do mature broccoli plants. That means that a 1-ounce ($\frac{1}{3}$ cup [28 g]) serving of broccoli sprouts will deliver roughly the same level of cancer-fighting compounds as would more than a pound (455 g) of broccoli.

Broccoli Sprouts: Good for the Gut

Broccoli sprouts have anticancer activity, are good for the heart (they may help lower total cholesterol, LDL ["bad"] cholesterol, and triglyceride levels), and may even benefit those with diabetes (eating sprouts may help improve blood sugar and insulin levels). But many people are surprised to learn that broccoli sprouts are also good for the gut.

Researchers have found that the cancer-fighting compound sulforaphane is also a powerful protector of the digestive tract. This compound triggers the cells in the gut to produce enzymes that protect against inflammation, DNA-damaging chemicals, and oxidative damage. Sulforaphane also appears to act as an antibiotic against certain harmful bacteria like *Helicobacter pylori*, which has been linked to gastritis (inflammation of the stomach), ulcers, and stomach cancer.

In a study published in 2009, researchers in Tokyo looked at the effects of a diet supplemented with broccoli or alfalfa sprouts in forty-eight patients infected with *H. pylori*. After eight weeks, they found that those who consumed 70 grams (about 2½ ounces) of broccoli sprouts daily had significant reductions in markers of inflammation and *H. pylori* infection (a similar intake of alfalfa sprouts had no such effects). Interestingly, two months after subjects stopped consuming the broccoli sprouts, those markers went back to their previous levels.

PUTTING IT INTO PRACTICE

Broccoli sprouts have a pleasing, peppery flavor and a few ounces (28 to 55 grams) added to salads, vegetable wraps, and veggie burgers are a great way to get a boost of flavor and nutrition. They are readily available at supermarkets and health food stores and can also be grown at home (see Resources, page 215, for more information).

Like other raw fruits and vegetables, sprouts carry a risk of food-borne illness. Because the seeds require a warm, moist environment for sprouting, it makes them an ideal breeding ground for bacteria. As a result, the U.S. Food and Drug Administration advises that children, the elderly, pregnant women, and those with impaired immune systems avoid eating raw or lightly cooked sprouts (particularly onion, alfalfa, clover, radish, and mung bean). It also recommends that everyone cook sprouts thoroughly and ask that sprouts not be added to your food when eating out.

If you choose to eat raw broccoli sprouts, there are a few things that you can do to minimize the risk of contamination. Buy fresh sprouts (or seeds) from reputable producers that have an International Sprout Growers Association (ISGA)–certified seal, which means that they follow guidelines to minimize risk of contamination and are certified by a third party. Fresh broccoli sprouts should also be just that: fresh. Avoid sprouts that are brown, slimy, odorous, or past their expiration date and keep sprouts refrigerated at all times. And as with all fruits and vegetables, wash thoroughly before consuming. Washing produce before eating, cutting, or cooking helps rid the surface of dirt, bacteria, and other particles.

AVOCADO AND SPROUT-STUFFED TOMATOES

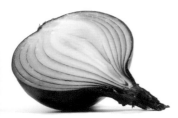

The broccoli sprouts in this recipe aren't just sprinkled on top of these little treats, but blended right into the thick and creamy filling. Stuffed cherry tomatoes are perfect bite-size snacks, but if you are looking for a more substantial side dish, you can hollow out and fill two or three vine-ripened tomatoes.

1 pint (300 g) cherry tomatoes
1 avocado, peeled and pitted
½ cup (17 g) plus ¼ cup (8 g) packed broccoli sprouts, divided
1 tablespoon (15 ml) freshly squeezed lime juice
¼ teaspoon sea salt
Pinch of garlic powder
2 tablespoons (20 g) diced red onion

Slice off the top of the cherry tomatoes and gently scoop out the inner pulp. Turn the tomatoes upside down on a paper towel to drain. Blend the avocado, ½ cup (17 g) of the broccoli sprouts, and the lime juice, sea salt, and garlic powder in a food processor until smooth and creamy. Transfer the filling to a small bowl and stir in the red onion. Spoon or pipe the filling into the tomatoes and garnish with the remaining ¼ cup (8 g) of broccoli sprouts.

Yield: 40 to 50 stuffed tomatoes

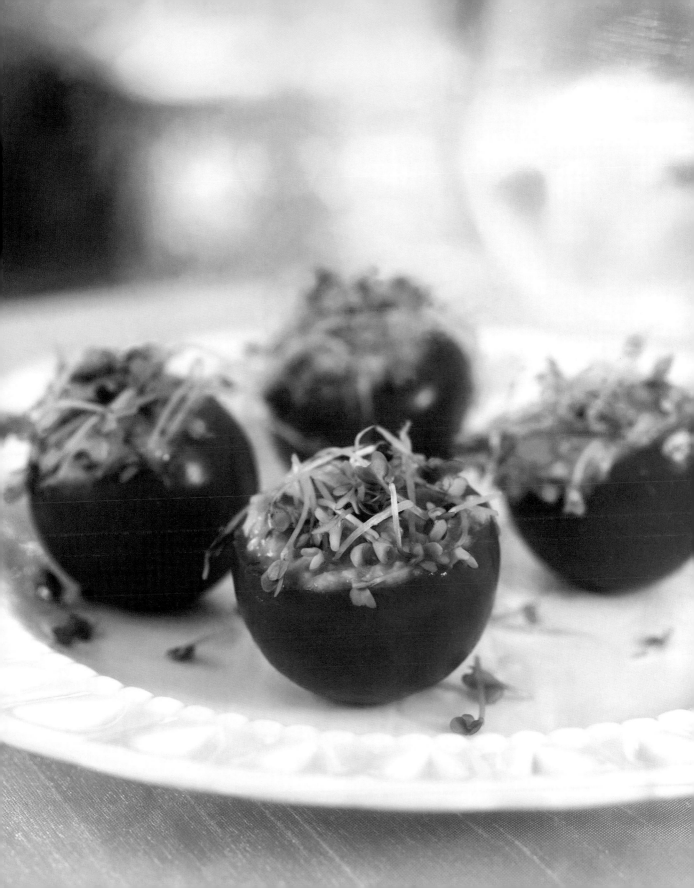

DANDELION GREENS
Liver-Loving Super Weed

SPOTLIGHT: VITAMIN K

Vitamin K is a fat-soluble vitamin that is abundant in leafy greens. It helps regulate blood clotting and maintains strong bones. Researchers have found that women who get at least 110 micrograms of vitamin K (the amount in a quarter-cup, or 14 grams, of dandelion or other leafy greens) are 30 percent less likely to have a hip fracture than are women who consume less. In fact, those who eat a serving of leafy greens each day (one serving equals 1 cup [55 g] of fresh greens or ½ cup [53 g] of cooked greens) cut their risk of hip fracture by 50 percent compared with those who eat leafy greens only once a week.

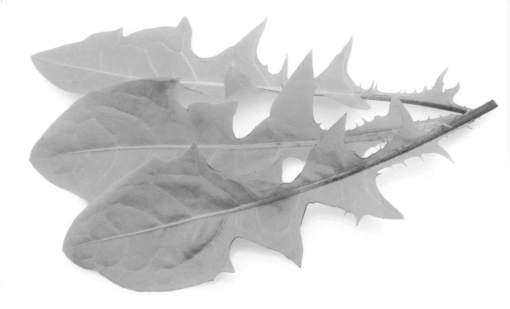

Dandelions (*Taraxacum officinale*) are perennial weeds of the Asteracaea family, which includes daisies, asters, and sunflowers. During the spring and summer months, they are often found dotting the lush green landscape with their vibrant yellow flowers. Although dandelions are often thought of as pesky weeds, they are actually a rich source of nutrients with potent antioxidant and anti-inflammatory properties. My wise grandmother would often pick young dandelion leaves right from the ground and toss them into salads. Dandelions—including their leaves and roots—have a long history of use in food and medicine, and researchers are discovering today that the dandelion is a potent health-promoting and disease-fighting food worthy of status higher than that of a common weed.

Packed with Bone-Building Calcium and Vitamin K

Dandelion leaves are edible greens that are rich in vitamins, minerals, antioxidants, and phytochemicals. A few handfuls of these fresh, chopped greens—around 3 cups [165 g]—tossed into a soup or smoothie deliver nearly 5 grams of protein (almost as much as the 7 grams in an egg) and about 6 grams of dietary fiber (almost a quarter of your daily needs).

A cup (55 g) of raw, chopped dandelion greens contains more than 100 milligrams of calcium (about one-third of the calcium in a cup of milk) along with nearly 2 milligrams of iron. Dandelion greens are also high in vitamins A and K, the latter of which is important for building strong bones. In fact, 1 cup (55 g) of fresh greens contains more than 400 micrograms of vitamin K—an impressive 350 to 475 percent of your daily needs.

Dandelion Greens Help Protect Against Toxins

Dandelion greens are rich in heart-protecting and cancer-fighting carotenoids and polyphenols. Eating dandelion leaves may help improve your blood lipids by lowering total and LDL ("bad") cholesterol levels while increasing HDL ("good") cholesterol levels—important factors in heart disease. Researchers have also found that the compounds in dandelion leaves can help stop the growth and proliferation of certain cancer cells, including those of the breast and prostate. And although these compounds can selectively target cancer cells, they appear to have a protective effect on other cells of the body, including those of the brain, liver, and blood vessels.

Studies have also shown that the antioxidants in dandelion leaves protect the liver against viruses like hepatitis and from injuries resulting from exposure to acetaminophen or other liver toxins. In a study published in 2012, researchers looked at the effects of dandelion leaf extracts in mice with acetaminophen-induced liver toxicity. Although acetaminophen is a common over-the-counter pain reliever, excess, long-term, or improper use may also cause liver problems. In the study, researchers found that dandelion leaf extracts helped prevent some of the adverse effects of acetaminophen on the liver, including tissue changes, increases in liver enzymes associated with liver dysfunction, and increases in certain markers of oxidative stress.

PUTTING IT INTO PRACTICE

Mildly bitter dandelion greens appear in the wild from early spring until the end of summer. You can pick the young leaves directly from the plant, but preferably before the yellow flower has bloomed, as the leaves turn tougher and more bitter after blooming. Dandelion greens are also cultivated and available year-round in most supermarkets. Choose greens that are fresh, tender-crisp, and with a stalk about the size of a pencil. Wrap them in a damp paper towel and store in a plastic bag in the refrigerator. Although dandelion greens will last up to one week in the fridge, use them within a day or two of purchase as they become more bitter with age.

Fresh dandelion greens can be added to salads, blended in smoothies, or juiced. You can also sauté or steam them as you would any leafy green vegetable. Try adding at least one serving of leafy greens—including dandelion greens—to your daily diet for a boost of antioxidants, fiber, and bone-building nutrients like calcium and vitamin K.

GARLICKY DANDELION GREENS AND BEANS

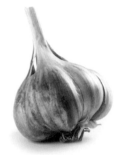

This recipe combines dandelion greens with cooked and raw garlic, for flavor and health. Cooking garlic weakens the activity of allicin, one of its cancer-fighting, immune-boosting compounds. But combining a small amount of raw garlic with greens and beans at the end of cooking infuses this dish with extra flavor and boosts its beneficial compounds.

3 cloves garlic, divided

1 large bunch dandelion greens

2 tablespoons (28 ml) extra-virgin olive oil
  Several pinches of red pepper flakes

1 cup (256 g) cooked or canned cannellini beans (white kidney beans) (drain and rinse, if canned)

3 tablespoons (27 g) raw pine nuts
  Sea salt and freshly ground pepper, to taste

Yield: 2 to 3 servings

Crush the garlic and set aside to rest at room temperature. Trim the stems off the dandelion greens and slice the leaves crosswise into bite-size pieces. Drizzle a large skillet with the olive oil, add 2 cloves worth of the crushed garlic and the red pepper flakes, and stir over medium heat until the garlic turns golden, 1 to 2 minutes. Add the greens to the skillet and toss with the oil and garlic to coat. Continue tossing the greens until they just begin to wilt, 1 to 2 minutes. Remove from the heat, add the beans, pine nuts, remaining crushed garlic, and salt and pepper to taste, and toss. Transfer to a serving dish and serve warm or at room temperature.

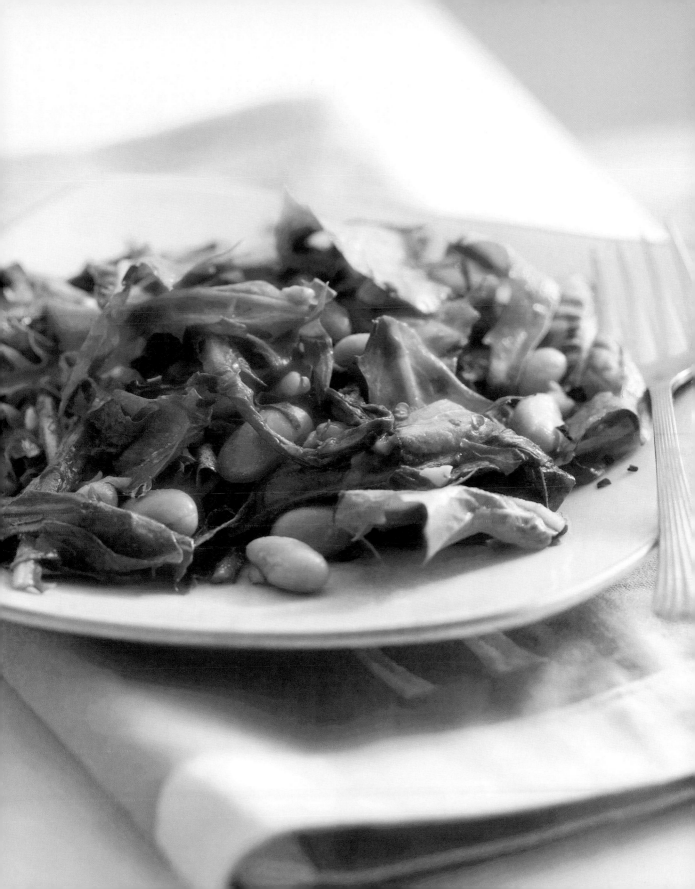

KALE
King of Greens

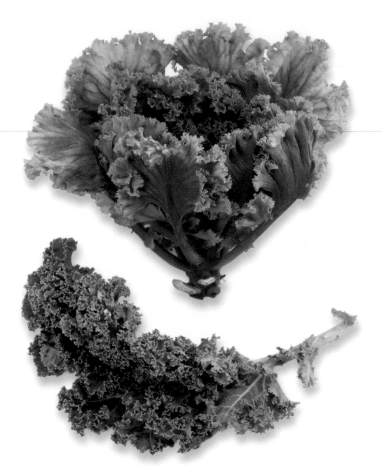

DID YOU KNOW?

The only way to activate the enzymes in kale—the ones responsible for converting its glucosinolates to active anticancer compounds—is to break down the tough cellular walls of the kale leaf. To do this, chop and chew or juice, blend, and sip your way to good health with a raw kale salad or kale-based juice or smoothie.

Kale is a powerhouse of health- promoting nutrients and cancer-fighting phytochemicals. A member of the Brassica family, which includes cruciferous vegetables like broccoli, cabbage, Brussels sprouts, and leafy greens like collard, mustard, and turnip greens, kale is a superfood for super health. Whether you juice it, blend it, wilt it, or bake it into a chip (yes, a kale chip!), this super green supports everything from healthy eyes and strong bones to preventing chronic disease.

Rich in Clot-Busting and Bone-Building Vitamin K

Kale boasts a wealth of important nutrients, including vitamins A and C and minerals like iron and calcium. One cup (67 g) of raw chopped kale meets more than 100 percent of your daily vitamin A needs, about 90 percent of your vitamin C needs, and a whopping 450 to 600 percent of your vitamin K needs—with nearly 550 milligrams per cup (67 g). Your body needs adequate vitamin K each and every day for good health. Vitamin K helps regulate blood clotting and maintain strong bones. And eating foods rich in this vitamin may also reduce your risk of cancer. Researchers have found that an ongoing deficiency of vitamin K is a risk factor for cancer, osteoporosis, and atherosclerosis (hardening of the arteries)—three good reasons to enjoy more of this and other leafy greens.

Kale's Cancer-Fighting Phytochemicals

Kale is also a rich source of numerous phytochemicals, including carotenoids and glucosinolates, sulfur-containing compounds that give it and other cruciferous vegetables their somewhat pungent odor and bitter taste. But these compounds are also important for good health. In the body, glucosinolates are converted into active compounds, including isothiocyanates (like sulforophane) and indoles (like indole-3-carbonyl). Researchers have found that these compounds help bind to and eliminate substances in the body that can cause DNA damage and cancer, and may also stop the growth and spreading of certain cancer cells, including those of the colon, stomach, and lungs. And because some of these compounds affect hormonal activities in the body, they may also help prevent hormone-sensitive breast and prostate cancers. Indeed, several population studies have found that higher intakes of cruciferous vegetables like kale—from 2 ounces (55 g) per day to three servings per week—are associated with a lower risk of certain cancers.

PUTTING IT INTO PRACTICE

Kale is available year-round, though its peak season is from winter through early spring. As with dandelion greens, look for smaller leaves, as they tend to have a milder flavor than larger ones. And try to use kale (and other greens) within a day or two of purchase; the longer they are stored, the more bitter they will become. To store kale, simply wrap it in a damp paper towel, place in a plastic bag, and refrigerate.

Kale makes a great addition to juices and smoothies. Try using two to three stalks of kale per juice along with other vegetables (like cucumbers and celery), herbs and spices (like fresh cilantro, parsley, or ginger), and a small amount of fruit (like lemons, limes, or an apple for added sweetness). You can also blend kale: simply trim off the hard stalk and toss a handful or two into any smoothie. Kale can be steamed or wilted (add nuts, seeds, or beans for a complete meal); tossed into soups, pasta, or vegetable dishes; or baked into kale chips. You can also enjoy raw kale in a salad like the recipe that follows.

MASSAGED KALE SALAD

SUPERFOOD KITCHEN TIP: EAT MORE (RAW) KALE

When you cook kale, you destroy the enzymes that help convert its glucosinolates into the active, cancer-fighting compounds your body needs. Fortunately, when that happens, the beneficial bacteria in your colon will step up and help produce those compounds. Unfortunately, the bacteria in your gut are not as efficient as the enzymes in making this conversion. So although you may enjoy steamed or wilted kale from time to time (I certainly do), try eating—or drinking—more raw kale for optimal levels of these cancer-fighting compounds. You can juice it, blend it, or make an uncooked massaged salad like the recipe in this section.

Gently massaging tough kale leaves with a blend of salt, lemon juice, and olive oil helps soften them and bring out their flavor. I like to top this salad with sprouted and salted pumpkin and sunflower seeds for an extra crunch and flavor, but you can use plain raw or roasted seeds as well.

1 large bunch kale

¼ teaspoon sea salt

1 tablespoon (15 ml) extra-virgin olive oil

1 tablespoon (15 ml) freshly squeezed lemon juice

¼ medium-size red onion, sliced thinly

½ avocado, peeled, pitted, and chopped

½ cup (120 g) cooked or canned chickpeas (garbanzo beans) (drain and rinse, if canned)

1 tablespoon (7 g) sprouted and salted pumpkin seeds

1 tablespoon (7 g) sprouted and salted sunflower seeds

1 tablespoon (8 g) hemp seeds

Freshly ground pepper

Remove and discard the tough stems from the kale and slice the leaves crosswise into thin ribbons. Place the kale leaves in a large serving bowl and add the salt, olive oil, and lemon juice. Massage the kale with your fingertips until it starts to soften, 2 to 3 minutes. Add the remaining ingredients to the bowl, toss to combine, and serve.

Yield: 4 to 6 servings (depending on type of kale used)

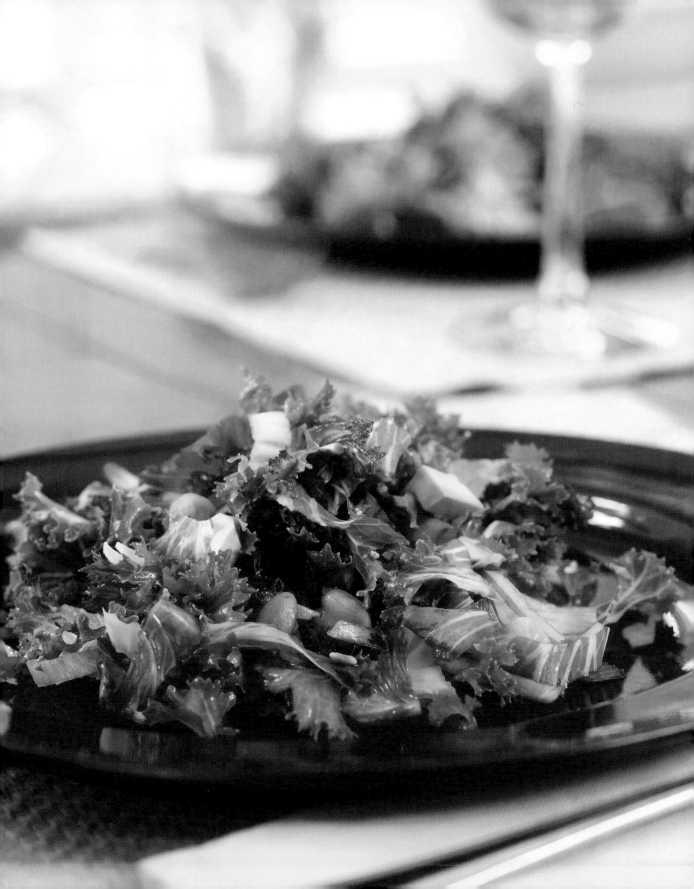

SPINACH
Super Green for Beginners

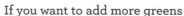

If you want to add more greens to your diet, spinach (*Spinacia oleracea*) is one of the simplest to start working with. Milder tasting than other leafy greens, spinach is a pleasing addition—in both flavor and nutrition—to nearly any diet. This superstar is packed with vitamins, minerals, antioxidants, and phyto-chemicals that help age-proof your brain, protect your heart, prevent cancer, and keep your eyes healthy. In fact, calorie for calorie, spinach has more nutrients than any other food, making it a top super green for optimal health.

Spinach is Rich in Blood-Building Iron

One cup (30 g) of fresh spinach contains more than 140 micrograms of immune-boosting vitamin A (15 to 20 percent of your daily needs) and nearly 150 micrograms of bone-building vitamin K (125 to 160 percent of your needs). And tossing a bunch of fresh spinach into your next smoothie will deliver about 9 milligrams of iron—more than 100 percent of the recommended dietary allowance for men and about

50 percent for most women. Spinach also contains numerous heart-healthy and cancer-fighting phytochemicals, including flavonoids and carotenoids like beta-carotene, lutein, and zeaxanthin, the latter two of which help prevent age-related eye diseases such as macular degeneration and cataracts.

Spinach May Reduce Risk of Heart Disease and Diabetes

Researchers have found that spinach may help lower the risk of high blood pressure and atherosclerosis (hardening of the arteries). And spinach, along with other leafy greens, may also decrease the risk of diabetes. In a review published in 2010, British researchers found that individuals who consumed 1.35 daily servings of leafy greens—1 to 2 cups (30 to 60 g) raw, or ½ to 1 cup (90 to 180 g) cooked—cut their risk of type 2 diabetes by 14 percent compared to those who consumed less than a quarter-serving. They attributed this effect to the combination of antioxidant nutrients and phytochemicals in leafy greens like spinach, including vitamin C, beta-carotene, folate, and polyphenols like flavonoids. Researchers also noted that spinach and other leafy greens are a good source of magnesium, a nutrient associated with a reduced risk of diabetes, and contain small amounts of alpha-linolenic acid, an omega-3 fatty acid found in the outer layer of cells that helps maintain insulin sensitivity.

Spinach Boasts Cancer-Combating Glycolipids

Spinach contains beneficial glycolipids, which are anticancer, antitumor compounds also found in beans and peas, leafy greens (like kale and parsley), and vegetables (like asparagus, broccoli, Brussels sprouts, bell peppers, and pumpkins, among others). These compounds appear to prevent the DNA in cancer cells from replicating. Indeed, researchers have found that glycolipid-rich extracts of spinach may prevent the growth of certain cancers, including those of the skin, prostate, colon, and cervix. A study published in 2008 found that mice who consumed oral doses of a glycolipid fraction of spinach for two weeks reduced their volume of colon tumors by more than 50 percent.

PUTTING IT INTO PRACTICE

The mild flavor of spinach makes it a great introduction to leafy greens for those who are new to them. It is most commonly available in the spring and fall months, as it grows best in cooler temperatures. Look for leaves that have a vibrant green color and avoid those that are pale green, yellow, slimy, or wilted. You can wrap fresh spinach in a damp paper towel and store it in a plastic bag in the refrigerator, where it will last for about three or four days.

Raw spinach can be tossed into smoothies or used alone or in combination with other greens to create raw salads. You can also add spinach to soups, casseroles, or pasta dishes to boost the nutrients in your cooked dishes. Spinach can also be gently steamed or sautéed and enjoyed alone or seasoned with crushed garlic, lemon juice, and extra-virgin olive oil, and sprinkled with nuts like slivered almonds, walnuts, or pine nuts. In fact, the healthy fats in nuts and olive oil will improve the absorption of the carotenoids and other fat-soluble compounds in this super green.

LUSCIOUS CASHEW CREAM AND SPINACH SOUP

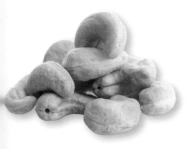

This simple soup combines a base of vegetable broth and cashew cream with 2 pounds (910 g) of fresh, iron-rich spinach. I love it as is, but if you want to add a subtle "cheesy" flavor to your bowl of soup—and boost of vitamin B_{12}—try sprinkling some nutritional yeast on top.

2 tablespoons (28 ml) extra-virgin olive oil

2 medium-size onions, chopped finely

4 cups (950 ml) vegetable stock

2 pounds (910 g) fresh spinach, stems removed and leaves chopped coarsely

½ cup (70 g) raw cashews, soaked for 6 to 8 hours

½ cup (120 ml) water

Several pinches of ground nutmeg

Sea salt and freshly ground pepper, to taste

Several pinches of nutritional yeast (optional)

Heat the oil in a large pot over medium heat. Add the onions and sauté until they are soft, 3 to 5 minutes. Add the vegetable stock to the pot and bring to a boil. Stir in the spinach, reduce the heat, and simmer, covered, for 15 to 20 minutes.

While the soup is simmering, drain and rinse the cashews and place them in a high-speed blender with ½ cup (120 ml) of water. Blend at high speed until smooth and creamy. Set aside.

When the soup has completed simmering, remove from the heat and stir in the cashew cream and nutmeg. Season with salt and pepper, to taste. Serve warm and top with a sprinkle of nutritional yeast, if desired.

Yield: 6 to 8 servings

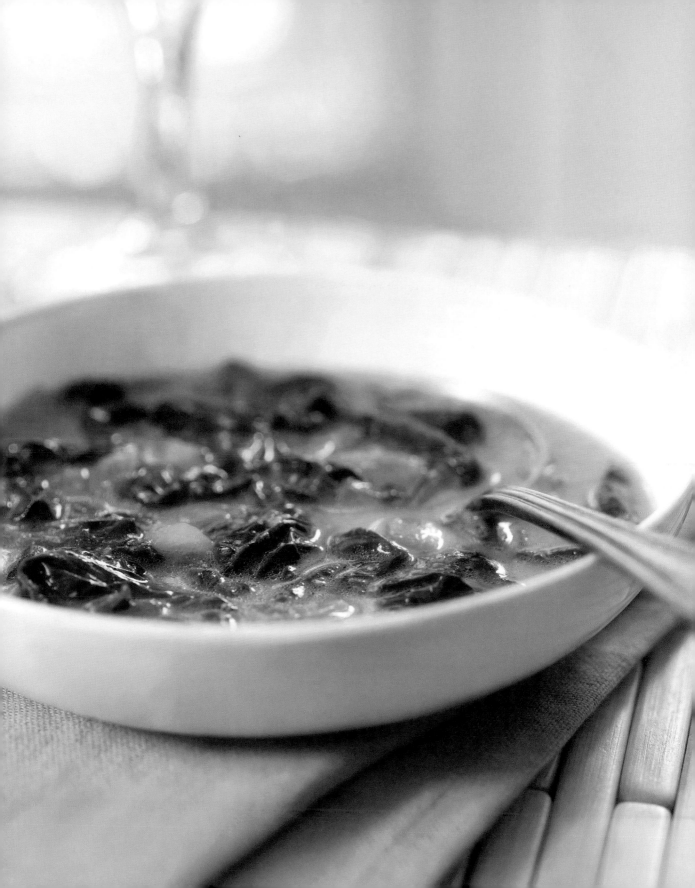

CHLORELLA
Iron-Rich Super Algae

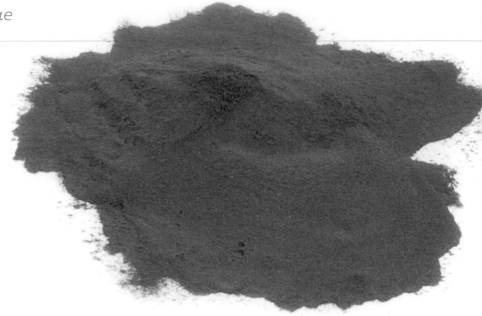

SPOTLIGHT: IRON

Iron is an essential mineral that helps make several important proteins in the body, including hemoglobin and myoglobin, which help transport oxygen to the body's tissues. You need an appropriate balance of iron in your body—too little may cause anemia and too much may be toxic—and although your body stocks iron, it loses about 10 percent of its stores each day. The good news is that you can get all the iron you need by consuming a variety of plant foods. In addition to chlorella, good sources include grains, legumes (beans, peas, and lentils), nuts, seeds, and leafy greens. Vitamin C helps increase the bioavailability of iron from plant foods—so citrus, camu camu berries, sea buckthorn berries, strawberries, and bell peppers are all great complements to iron-rich plant foods.

Chlorella is a microscopic, freshwater algae that is sometimes referred to as green algae or sun chlorella. Most of the chlorella available in the United States today is cultivated in Japan and Taiwan, the two most common varieties being *Chlorella pyrenoidosa* and *Chlorella vulgaris*. Chlorella has been touted as a superfood, with benefits ranging from preventing cancer and boosting immunity to increasing energy and detoxifying the body. Although there are few studies to support these claims, a growing body of research suggests that chlorella may give your health a boost.

Blood-Building Algae

Chlorella is rich in a variety of nutrients, including the energy-enhancing and stress-reducing B-vitamins, amino acids, and bone- and blood-building minerals like magnesium and iron. In fact, chlorella contains about 1.2 milligrams of iron per gram, meaning that a small amount—just 1 teaspoon—delivers about 3.6 milligrams of iron (20 to nearly 50 percent of the average adult's daily iron needs and about 13 percent of women's needs during pregnancy). And researchers have found that supplementing the diet with chlorella, particularly throughout pregnancy, may help prevent anemia.

In a study published in 2010, researchers from Japan found that women who supplemented daily with 6 grams of chlorella (about 2 teaspoons, containing 7.2 milligrams of iron) throughout pregnancy—beginning at twelve to eighteen weeks' gestation—had significantly lower rates of anemia in their second and third trimesters compared to those who did not supplement with chlorella. The study group was also less likely to suffer from edema (swelling in body tissues) and proteinuria (a condition in which urine contains abnormal amounts of protein)—both of which are associated with high blood pressure during pregnancy.

Toxin-Binding Superfood

Researchers have found that chlorella has strong antioxidant and anti-inflammatory effects that may play a positive role in the prevention and treatment of chronic disease. Chlorella may help reduce triglyceride, total cholesterol, and LDL ("bad") cholesterol levels, and may help improve blood pressure in those with mild to moderate hypertension. A few studies also suggest that chlorella can boost the immune system and inhibit the growth and proliferation of certain cancer cells.

Additionally, chlorella is thought to help prevent the accumulation of toxins—like heavy metals and pesticides—in the body by binding with and preventing their absorption in the gut. In a study published in 2005, mice fed a 10 percent, chlorella-enriched diet over five weeks excreted more dioxin (a toxic chemical that forms as a by-product during the manufacturing of chlorine-containing chemicals and plastics) than those fed a control diet. They also accumulated significantly lower levels of dioxin in their liver compared to those fed a 10 percent spinach-enriched or control diet. And researchers have seen similar effects in humans.

In a study published in 2005, researchers found that women who supplemented with chlorella during pregnancy had 30 percent lower levels of dioxins in their breast milk compared to the control group. And in a study published in the *Journal of Medicinal Food* in 2007, women who supplemented with chlorella during pregnancy not only had lower levels of toxins in their breast milk, but had increased levels of IgA (an important antibody)—both of which benefit nursing infants.

PUTTING IT INTO PRACTICE

Chlorella is one of the few superfoods in this book that is available only in supplement form, typically as a tablet, liquid extract, granule, or powder. Liquids, granules, and powders can be added to freshly pressed juices and smoothies. Green chlorella–containing powders also provide a convenient way to "drink" your greens when you may not have access to fresh juices or smoothies; simply add a scoop to bottled juice or water while traveling.

If you choose to consume chlorella, purchase products from a reputable company that can verify its products have been standardized and tested for purity. Also discuss any supplements you are taking with your health-care provider, especially if you are a woman who is pregnant or breastfeeding.

SUPER BERRY AND GREENS SMOOTHIE

The sweet flavor of the berries is a nice complement to the greens in this drink—making it a perfect "green" smoothie for beginners (you can hardly taste the greens). Although this recipe calls for a scoop of chlorella powder, you can use any green powder or leafy greens you have on hand. I often toss in a large handful of kale, spinach, or dandelion greens—all superfoods in their own right.

1½ cups (355 ml) filtered water

1 medium-size banana, sliced

1 packet (3½ ounces, or 100 g) frozen açai pulp

1 cup (155 g) frozen blueberries

1 tablespoon (14 g) coconut oil

1 vanilla bean, scraped, or 1 teaspoon pure vanilla extract

1 serving-size scoop (per manufacturer) chlorella-containing green powder

Combine all the ingredients in a high-speed blender and blend until smooth.

Yield: 2 servings

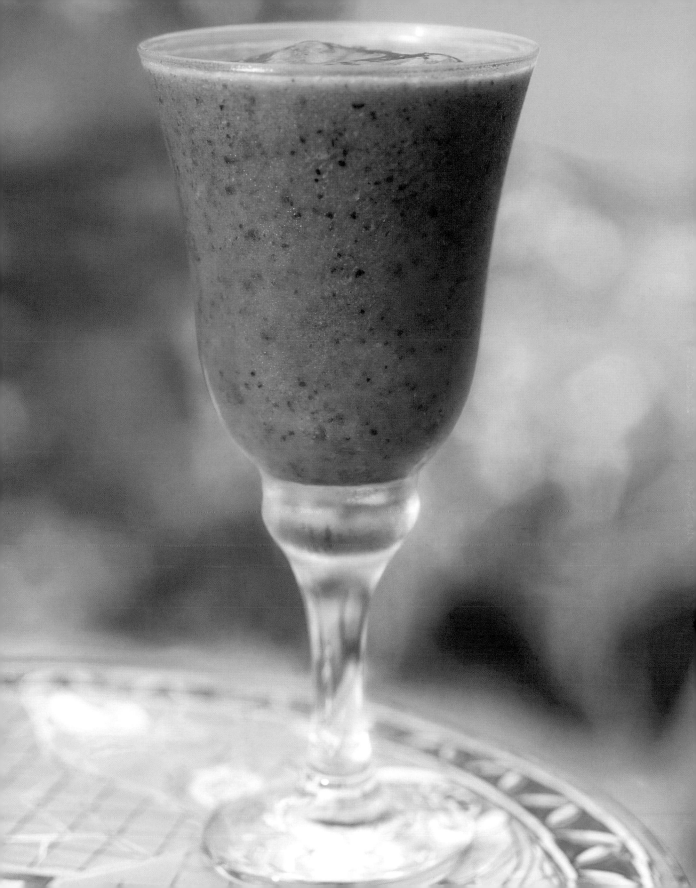

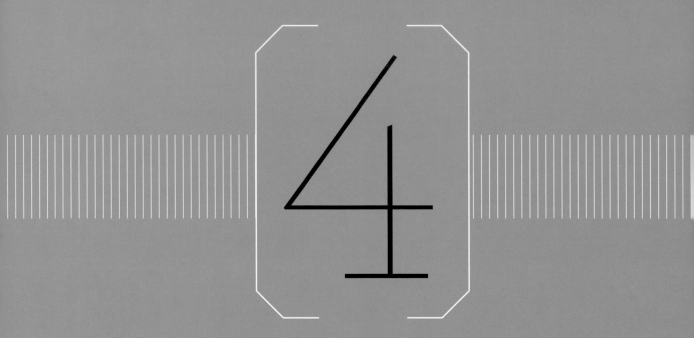

SUPER VEGETABLES AND LEGUMES

*Carob, Maca, Mesquite, Mushrooms,
Sea Vegetables, Pumpkin, Yacon*

These super-nutritious vegetable and legumes contain active compounds to help strengthen and support your body. Carob calms the gut, maca helps build resistance to stress, and sea vegetables contain the natural iodine necessary to support your thyroid. And these modern-day superfoods—including cancer-fighting mushrooms and pumpkin and blood sugar–friendly carob, mesquite, and yacon—may also help fend off modern-day conditions like heart disease, cancer, and diabetes.

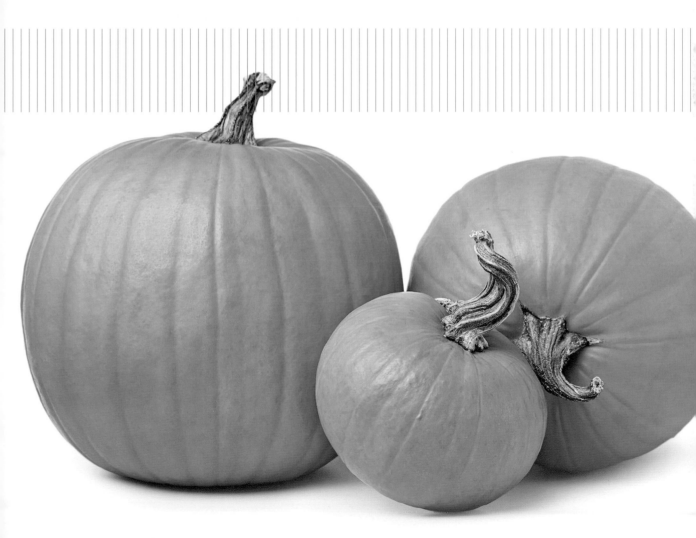

CAROB
Antioxidant-Rich Chocolate Alternative

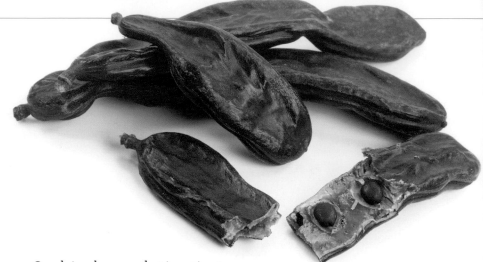

SPOTLIGHT: DIETARY FIBER

Dietary fiber is the carbohydrate portion of plant foods that your body cannot digest and absorb, and it is essential for good health. There are two forms of dietary fiber: soluble and insoluble. Soluble fiber is found in certain fruits and vegetables, oats, barley, legumes (beans, peas, lentils), and seeds; it has been shown to lower blood sugar and cholesterol levels. Insoluble fiber is found in most vegetables, nuts, and wheat; it adds bulk to the stool and helps speed the passage of food through the digestive tract. Older children, adolescents, and adults should aim to consume 25 to 35 grams of dietary fiber each day, but according to the National Institutes of Health, the average American meets less than half of this recommendation.

Carob is a legume that is native to the Mediterranean and originates from the pods of the carob tree (*Ceratonia siliqua*). Edible carob pods contain both an inner pulp and seeds, which can be dried, roasted, and ground into a nutrient- and fiber-rich powder. Carob powder is often used in place of cocoa powder, particularly by those looking for a stimulant-free alternative to chocolate. But even for those not seeking a chocolate substitute, carob is a tasty and nutritious addition to the diet. With a history of use going back more than four thousand years, carob is becoming a modern-day superfood that may help promote heart health, improve digestion, and even offer protection against cancer.

Calcium- and Fiber-Packed Pod

Carob is packed with numerous minerals, including magnesium, potassium, iron, and calcium.

One cup (128 g) of carob powder boasts around 350 milligrams of calcium—more than an equivalent serving of milk and nearly double that of cacao. Just 2 tablespoons (16 g) of carob powder—the amount you might add to a smoothie or cup of hot "chocolate"—meets about 5 percent of your daily calcium needs. In addition, carob is an excellent source of dietary fiber. Two tablespoons (16 g) of powder provide about 5 grams of fiber—an impressive 15 to 20 percent of your daily needs.

Like chocolate, carob contains numerous polyphenols with strong antioxidant properties that may benefit the heart. Studies have shown that carob may help lower total cholesterol, LDL ("bad") cholesterol, and triglycerides. And the polyphenols in carob may also play a role in cancer prevention. Some polyphenols, such as gallic acid, appear to have strong antioxidant and cytotoxic activities against cancer cells, including those of the cervix and colon.

Tannin-Rich Carob Soothes the Intestines

Traditionally, carob has been used in the treatment of diarrhea, and it is still recommended today for alleviating digestive upset, including reflux and irritable bowel syndrome. Carob eases diarrhea through its rich content of tannins, polyphenols that have an astringent-like quality that may help soothe the intestines. Mixing a tablespoon (8 g) of carob with applesauce, mashed banana, or other pureed fruit may offer relief from diarrhea or irritable bowel symptoms. In addition, several studies have found that the addition of carob bean gum (also called locust bean gum) to infant formulas helps reduce reflux and vomiting because of its thickening abilities.

PUTTING IT INTO PRACTICE

Carob is often used as a substitute for chocolate, though I find it has a unique flavor that is slightly sweeter (and milder, not bitter tasting) than chocolate. Carob can be purchased as a syrup, chip, or powder at most supermarkets and health food stores. Drizzle carob syrup over fruit for added sweetness or use it as a spread. You can use carob chips in place of chocolate chips in baked and raw desserts. Carob chips often have added sugar, fat, soy, and dairy, so be sure to read food labels. Vegan carob chips are a good nondairy option, but they are typically made with malted barley and are not suitable for those following a gluten-free diet.

Using raw or roasted carob powder is probably one of the simplest ways to enjoy the benefits of this superfood. Toss a tablespoon (8 g) or two of carob powder into a smoothie or use it to make a homemade "hot chocolate," which you can spice up with a little cinnamon, nutmeg, or cayenne. As a general rule, for one part cocoa substitute 1½ to 2 parts carob by weight or mix 3 tablespoons (24 g) of carob powder with 1 tablespoon (15 ml) of water per square of chocolate.

CAROB BARK

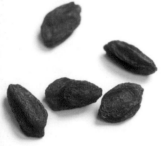

The combination of high-protein and fat-rich nuts and seeds along with naturally sweet and antioxidant-rich berries makes this a simple and delicious snack for sustained energy.

¾ cup carob powder (96 g)
½ cup (120 ml) water
3 tablespoons (42 g) coconut oil
1 tablespoon (20 g) pure maple syrup
½ teaspoon pure vanilla extract
  Pinch of sea salt
¼ cup (16 g) raw pumpkin seeds
¼ cup (25 g) raw cashews, chopped
¼ cup (23 g) goji berries
¼ cup (30 g) dried mulberries

Yield: 12 to 15 broken pieces

Combine the carob powder, water, and coconut oil in a saucepan over low heat. Stir continuously until the coconut oil has melted and the ingredients have combined into a thick paste, about 3 minutes. Remove from the heat, stir in the maple syrup, vanilla, and salt, and continue stirring until the mixture is smooth and creamy. Fold in the seeds, nuts, and berries, and spread evenly—about ½-inch (1.3 cm) thick—onto a waxed paper–lined baking dish. Freeze for about 1 hour or until the carob bark has completely hardened. Remove the bark from the waxed paper and cut or break into pieces. Keep refrigerated or freeze for long-term storage.

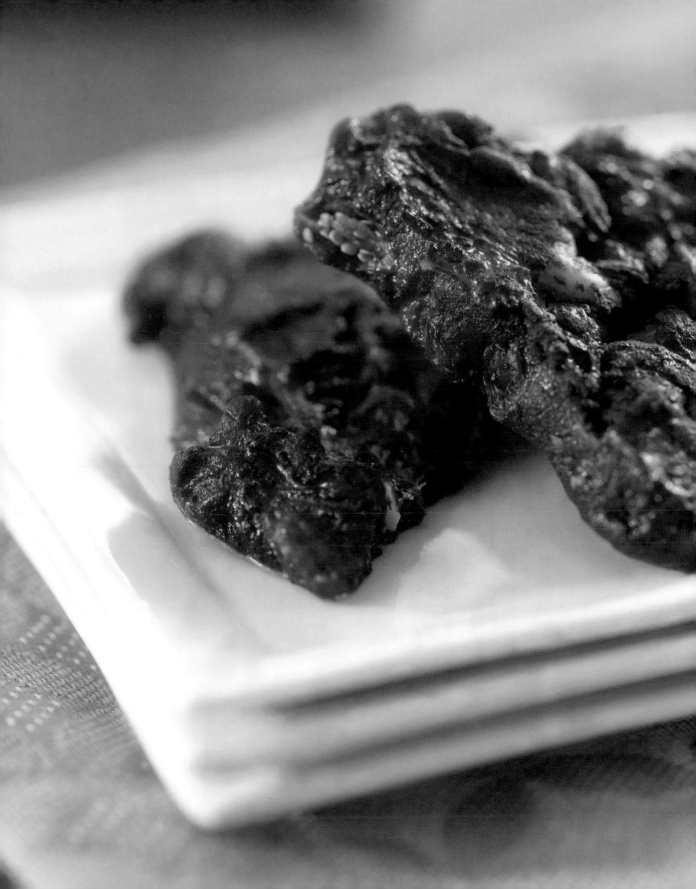

MACA
Super Adaptogenic Root

Maca contains phytosterols, plant-based compounds that inhibit the absorption of cholesterol and may even help lower total and LDL ("bad") cholesterol levels. Some studies have also found that higher intakes of phytosterols may decrease cancer risk. Phytosterols are found in maca and other plant foods, including wheat germ, vegetable oils (like olive and sesame oils), peanuts, almonds, and wheat bran.

Maca is an annual plant (*Lepidium meyenii*) that grows in the high elevations of the Andes. Native to Peru, it has been cultivated for thousands of years for its fleshy root, which has traditionally been used to increase stamina, reduce fatigue, boost libido, and enhance fertility. Reportedly, Incan warriors would often consume maca prior to battle for strength and stamina—though they were prohibited from using it after victory to protect women from the heightened sexual desires that might occur from its use. Indeed, there is a limited but growing body of research that is only beginning to unfold the potential benefits of maca and support some of its traditional uses. But if you are looking to enhance your overall well-being—and perhaps your sex life—this super root vegetable may be a welcome addition to your diet.

Stress-Busting Super Root

Maca has a diverse mix of vitamins, minerals, amino acids, and fats. A single teaspoon of raw maca powder boasts a modest gram each of fiber and protein, along with 2 percent each of your daily calcium and iron needs. It is also high in beneficial phytosterols and alkamides, compounds thought to strengthen and support the endocrine system, which regulates nearly every bodily process from your metabolism and mood to growth and sexual function.

Alkamide-rich maca is widely known as an adaptogen, which enhances the body's natural ability to respond or "adapt" to stress (for example, physical stress like intense exercise or mental stress like anxiety). Adaptogens strengthen the systems of the body—without overstimulating or inhibiting normal functions—and bring them back to a balanced state when outside stressors threaten to disrupt them. The alkamides in maca, in particular a group called macamides, are thought to be part of this support and responsible, at least in part, for maca's potential to enhance sexual function.

Superfood for Super Sex

A small number of animal studies over the past decade have found that maca may boost libido, improve sexual behavior, enhance the production of sperm, and increase fertility (this super root seems to help increase sperm count and motility). One study also found that maca supplementation reduced prostate size in rats with enlarged prostates.

In human studies, researchers have found that supplementing with maca root powder—in amounts ranging from 1½ to 3½ grams (1/3 to 2/3 teaspoon) daily—may improve energy, mood, libido, and fertility. In a study published in 2009, Italian researchers found that maca root powder—2.4 grams (½ teaspoon) administered over a twelve-week period—resulted in a small but significant improvement in sexual function and overall well-being in men with mild erectile dysfunction. And a study published in *Menopause* in 2008 found that postmenopausal women who received 3½ grams (2/3 teaspoon) of maca powder for six weeks had lower measures of sexual dysfunction and reduced anxiety and depression. Although treatment with maca in amounts of 1½ to 3½ grams (1/3 to 2/3 teaspoons) appears to offer some benefits regarding sexual function, studies have shown that those same amounts seem to have no measurable effects on hormone levels in men or women. Thus, the mechanism by which maca confers benefits remains unclear and certainly more research is needed to better understand the actions of this super root.

PUTTING IT INTO PRACTICE

Maca is most commonly available as a raw or gelatinized powder. I recommend using the raw powder, which has a unique malted flavor. It consists only of the maca root, which is dried at low temperatures and then ground. Maca powder is a delicious addition to smoothies and nut milks and can be incorporated into or sprinkled on desserts, snacks, and cereals. From the standpoint of flavor, it combines particularly well with coconut, cacao, and vanilla. I often roll chocolate truffles in maca powder, sprinkle it on raw cacao brownies, or add a scoop to homemade vanilla or chocolate nut milks. Adding a teaspoon or two of this powder into your favorite smoothies and desserts is a simple way to include this super root in your diet.

MACA PECAN ICE CREAM

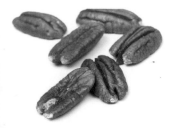

This maca and maple-flavored ice cream is a thick, rich, and creamy frozen treat. And the pecans not only add extra crunch and flavor to this dish, but a big boost of nutrients. Pecans are packed with more than nineteen different vitamins and minerals, heart-healthy unsaturated fats, and boast one of the highest levels of antioxidants of all nuts.

1 cup (140 g) raw cashews, soaked for 1 to 2 hours

½ cup (120 ml) water

⅔ cup (213 g) pure maple syrup

½ cup (113 g) coconut oil

1 tablespoon (15 g) raw maca powder

Pinch of sea salt

¼ cup (25 g) raw pecans, chopped

Yield: 4 servings

Drain and rinse the cashews. Blend the cashews and water until creamy. Add the maple syrup, coconut oil, maca powder, and salt and blend until smooth. Pour into an ice-cream maker and process per the manufacturer's instructions, gradually adding the pecans to the ice cream as it begins to thicken. Transfer the ice cream to a tightly lidded container and freeze.

If you do not have an ice-cream maker, simply pour the mixture into a glass dish, cover, and freeze. As the ice cream begins to thicken, stir in the pecans.

Keep frozen. Let stand at room temperature for a few minutes before serving to soften.

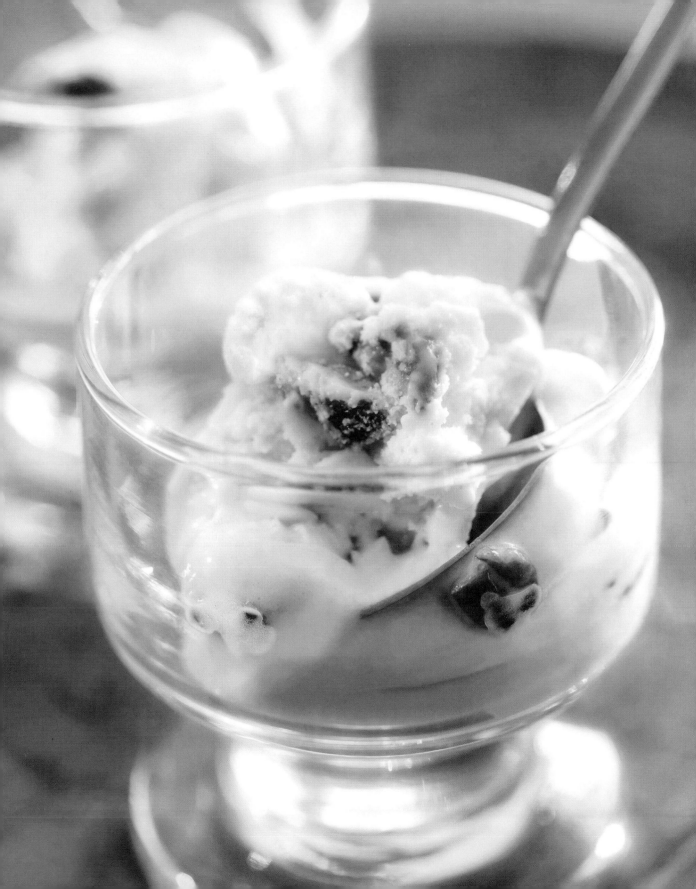

MESQUITE

Low-Glycemic-Index Super Legume

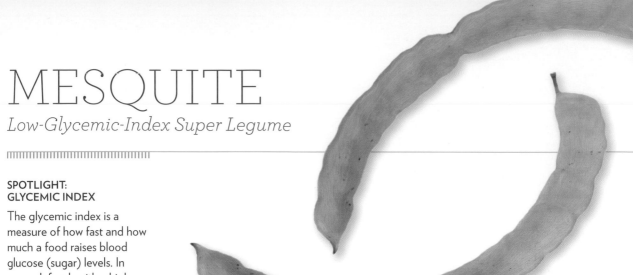

The glycemic index is a measure of how fast and how much a food raises blood glucose (sugar) levels. In general, foods with a high glycemic index (70 or more) will raise blood sugars more rapidly than do foods with a low glycemic index (55 or less). High-glycemic-index foods include pasta, bread, rice, and baked goods, whereas low-glycemic-index foods include most fruits, vegetables, and legumes like mesquite, which has a glycemic index of 25. You can choose low-glycemic-index foods more often to help better regulate your blood sugar—or even combine two groups of foods (for example, rice and beans)—to bring down the glycemic load of an entire meal.

Mesquite (mes-keet) is the edible pod of leguminous trees and shrubs (of the genus *Prosopis*) native to North and South America. Mesquite trees grow in harsh and dry desert regions that are not well tolerated by other crops; in fact, the plant is so hardy that it will continue to produce pods during droughts. Its durability is a likely factor in its role as a staple food for centuries of native peoples throughout the Americas. Today, mesquite is just beginning to gain popularity as a superfood. Unlike popular "mesquite seasonings" (which typically contain no mesquite), mesquite powder, made from the ground edible mesquite pods, is best known for its beneficial effect on blood sugars. Its sweet, smoky, molasses-like flavor makes it a welcome addition to many modern-day dishes.

Low-Glycemic-Index, Fiber-Rich Legume

Although mesquite tastes rather sweet, it is actually a low-glycemic-index food that will not cause a sharp rise in blood sugar when consumed. In a study published in 1990 in the *American Journal of Clinical Nutrition*, researchers reported that mesquite had one of the lowest glycemic index scores of traditional Pima Indian foods that included corn, lima beans, acorns, and teparies (twining beans). Mesquite is an excellent source of dietary fiber, which helps slow the digestion and release of sugars into the bloodstream. One tablespoon (14 g) of mesquite powder contains about 3 grams of dietary fiber—around 10 percent of your daily needs.

Mesquite may not only prevent blood sugars from rising but also help regulate them. In a study published in 2011, researchers looked at the effects of the dried and ground pods of honey mesquite (*Prosopis glandulosa*) in rats with type 1 diabetes. They found that treatment with mesquite over an eight-week period significantly increased insulin levels and significantly decreased blood sugar levels. They also found that treatment with mesquite boosted the beta cells of the pancreas—the cells responsible for producing and secreting insulin. Damage to these cells is characteristic of type 1 diabetes.

Mesquite May Improve Blood Pressure

In a cell study published in the *Journal of Medicinal Food* in 2009, researchers looked at the effects of an extract of algarrobo (*Prosopis pallida*), a type of mesquite native to South America, on enzymes involved in starch digestion and blood pressure regulation. They found that the mesquite extract actually blocked the activity of an enzyme responsible for converting starches to sugar—similar to the actions of alpha-glucosidase inhibitors (oral antidiabetic drugs that are used to control blood sugars). In addition, the extract also acted as an angiotensin-converting enzyme (ACE) inhibitor, preventing the body from producing angiotensin II, a substance that can cause blood vessels to narrow and release hormones that will raise your blood pressure. Perhaps mesquite will prove to be a natural regulator of blood pressure and blood sugar levels, though more studies are certainly needed.

PUTTING IT INTO PRACTICE

Mesquite powder is available at most supermarkets and health food stores. Look for products that contain only mesquite powder, which is created from the dried and ground edible mesquite pods. By contrast, products labeled "mesquite seasoning" typically contain a blend of spices, oils, additives, and flavorings—and no beneficial mesquite.

Because it has a naturally sweet, smoky, and molasses-like flavor, mesquite powder makes a nice addition to recipes incorporating vanilla or cacao, such as nut milks, ice creams, and other desserts. I also enjoy sprinkling it on roasted or grilled root vegetables like sweet potatoes and winter squash. Although it is hard to say exactly how much mesquite you would need to consume for its potential health benefits, a teaspoon or two of powder added to smoothies, nut milks, desserts, and roasted root vegetables will certainly give you a boost of flavor and nutrition.

MESQUITE SWEET POTATO HASH

This recipe was inspired by my mom's original recipe for potato pancakes. I substituted sweet potatoes for regular potatoes, added mesquite, and omitted the flour and egg. This hash is full of flavor and cancer-fighting carotenoids, vitamin C, and minerals like calcium, potassium, and magnesium. Enjoy as a breakfast or dinner side dish or toss with greens and beans for a complete meal.

2 large sweet potatoes, peeled and shredded (about 2 pounds, or 910 g)

½ medium-size onion, chopped finely

2 tablespoons (8 g) chopped fresh parsley

1 tablespoon (14 g) mesquite powder

1½ teaspoons sea salt

¼ teaspoon freshly ground pepper

Pinch of ground nutmeg

2 tablespoons (28 ml) grapeseed oil

In a large mixing bowl, combine all the ingredients except the grapeseed oil and mix well. Heat the grapeseed oil in a large skillet over medium heat. Add the sweet potato mixture to the skillet and sauté for 15 to 20 minutes until browned. Remove from the heat and serve warm.

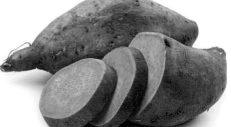

Yield: 5 to 6 servings

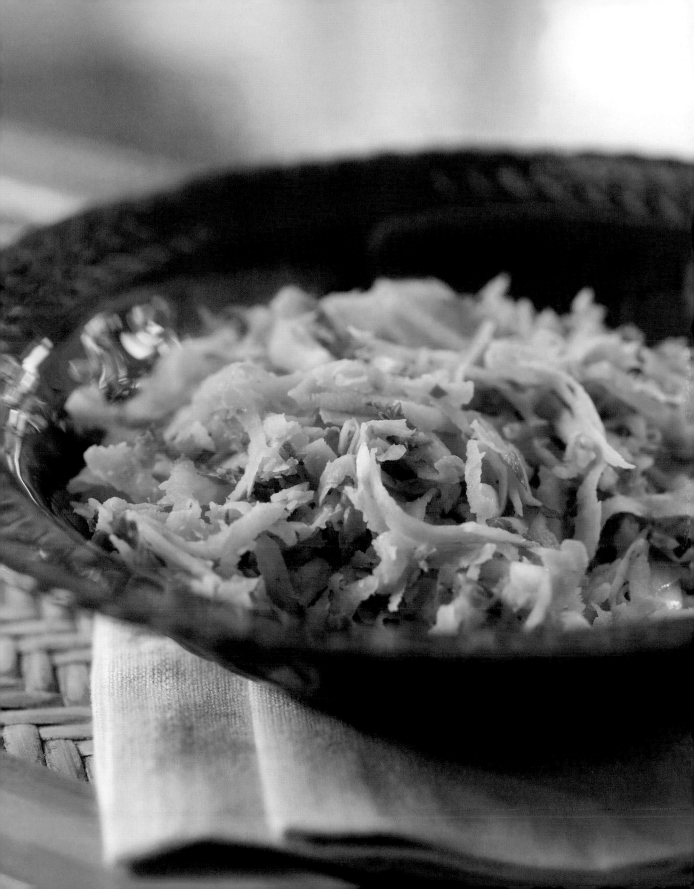

MUSHROOMS

Immune-Boosting, Cancer-Fighting Fungi

SPOTLIGHT: VITAMIN D

Mushrooms contain small and varying amounts of ergosterol, a precursor to vitamin D_2, and vitamin D. A fat-soluble hormone, vitamin D promotes calcium absorption in the gut; supports bone growth and mineralization; reduces inflammation; and helps the immune, muscular, and nervous systems. Adequate levels may even protect against autoimmune diseases, while deficiencies have been linked to an increased risk of bone fractures and cancer.

Although researchers have found that exposing mushrooms to UV light can boost their vitamin D content, most are still cultivated in the dark—so for now, I wouldn't look to mushrooms to meet your daily vitamin D needs.

Mushrooms are commonly categorized as vegetables in the nutrition world, but this superfood is technically a fungus. There are an estimated fourteen thousand different species of mushrooms, about three thousand of which are considered edible. They have been used for centuries for food and medicine, and today they are being recognized as a modern-day superfood. In fact, the authors of one 2012 review on mushrooms referred to them as "miniature pharmaceutical factories" because of their hundreds of health-promoting nutrients and compounds. These antioxidant-rich and anti-inflammatory fungi have strong immune-boosting, anticancer, antitumor, and antiviral properties. From common mushrooms like white button and portobello to more exotic varieties like maitake and shiitake, mushrooms are potent power foods that make a delicious and nutritious addition to your diet.

Number One Selenium Supplier

The nutrient and phytochemical content of mushrooms vary widely depending upon the variety of mushroom, the age of the mushroom, where it was grown, and how it was cultivated. But in general, mushrooms are a good source of important vitamins and minerals—like the B vitamins riboflavin and niacin and minerals like copper and potassium.

A single serving of mushrooms—about ½ cup (54 g) cooked—contains anywhere from 200 to 400 milligrams of potassium, a mineral that may help lower blood pressure and reduce the risk of stroke.

Mushrooms are also unusually high in selenium, a trace mineral with strong antioxidant and free radical–scavenging abilities. In fact, mushrooms contain more of this trace mineral than any other fruit or vegetable, and its intake has been associated with a reduced risk of certain cancers, including lung, prostate, and colon cancer. Cremini mushrooms contain one of the highest levels of selenium—about 22 grams per serving—which meets about 30 percent of your daily needs.

Mushrooms Boost the Immune System and Fight Cancer

Researchers have found that mushrooms contain numerous compounds—from polysaccharides and flavonoids to carotenoids and tocopherols—that may help stimulate the immune system and fight cancer. Shiitake mushrooms (*Lentinus edodes*) produce a compound called lentinan, a beta-glucan polysaccharide that helps boost the immune system and fight off infections—and cancer—by stimulating the activity of the body's white blood cells. Maitake mushrooms (*Grifola frondosa*) also contain polysaccharides with immune-boosting and cancer-fighting activities. Cell studies have shown that polysaccharide-rich extracts from maitake mushrooms prevent the growth and proliferation of certain cancer cells (like those of the stomach), triggering them to self-destruct. In addition, researchers have found that shiitake mushrooms may also help lower cholesterol levels, while maitake mushrooms may help regulate blood pressure and blood sugar levels.

Common varieties like cremini, portobello, and white button (*Agaricus bisporus*) are also powerful cancer-fighting fungi. In a study published in the *Journal of Nutrition*, researchers found that active compounds in white button mushrooms inhibit the actions of enzymes involved in estrogen production, which means that they may help prevent the development or progression of hormone-driven cancers like breast cancer.

PUTTING IT INTO PRACTICE

Mushrooms grow wild and are cultivated throughout the world, with top producers including China and the United States. White button mushrooms are the most commonly consumed mushrooms in the United States, though other common varieties, such as cremini and portobello, along with exotic varieties like shiitake, maitake, enoki, and oyster are becoming increasingly popular.

Look for both fresh and dried mushrooms at the supermarket. Fresh mushrooms should be stored in a paper bag in the refrigerator and should not be washed until use to prevent premature spoiling. Simply trim off the woody stem and scrub the caps gently using your fingers or a small mushroom brush.

From flavorful shiitake and portobello mushrooms to milder-tasting enoki and oyster mushrooms, adding a few servings of fungi to your weekly meals is easy. Mushrooms are great sautéed or grilled and added to stir-fries, salads, and pasta or simmered into soups for added flavor. I sometimes sauté and enjoy them alone with a little drizzle of olive oil and freshly ground salt and pepper. If you are looking for a meat-free alternative to the traditional hamburger or soy-based burger, enjoy the meaty texture of a portobello mushroom. No matter how you cook or serve them, aim for a few servings (one serving equals ½ cup [54 g] of cooked mushrooms) of these super fungi each week for a boost of immune-boosting and cancer-fighting compounds.

WALNUT AND PARSLEY PESTO STUFFED MUSHROOMS

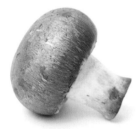

These baked mushrooms combine a few simple and healthful ingredients like omega-3 fatty-acid rich walnuts and immune-boosting garlic. The addition of nutritional yeast adds a mildly "cheesy" flavor—and boost of vitamin B_{12}—to these little treats.

1	cup (60 g) tightly packed fresh parsley
1	cup (100 g) raw walnuts
1	tablespoon (15 ml) freshly squeezed lemon juice
2	cloves garlic, crushed
2	tablespoons (12 g) nutritional yeast
6	tablespoons (90 ml) extra-virgin olive oil, divided
	Sea salt and freshly ground pepper, to taste
12 to 15	cremini mushrooms, stems removed

Yield: 12 to 15 mushrooms

Preheat the oven to 375°F (190°C, or gas mark 5). Place the parsley, walnuts, lemon juice, garlic, nutritional yeast, and 2 tablespoons (30 ml) of the olive oil in a food processor and pulse until coarsely chopped. Transfer to a small mixing bowl and add salt and pepper to taste.

Drizzle a 9 × 13-inch (23 × 33 cm) baking dish with 2 tablespoons (30 ml) of the olive oil. Fill the mushrooms and place, filled side up, on the baking dish. Drizzle the remaining 2 tablespoons (30 ml) of olive oil over the mushrooms. Bake for about 20 minutes until the mushrooms are soft and the filling is browned and heated through.

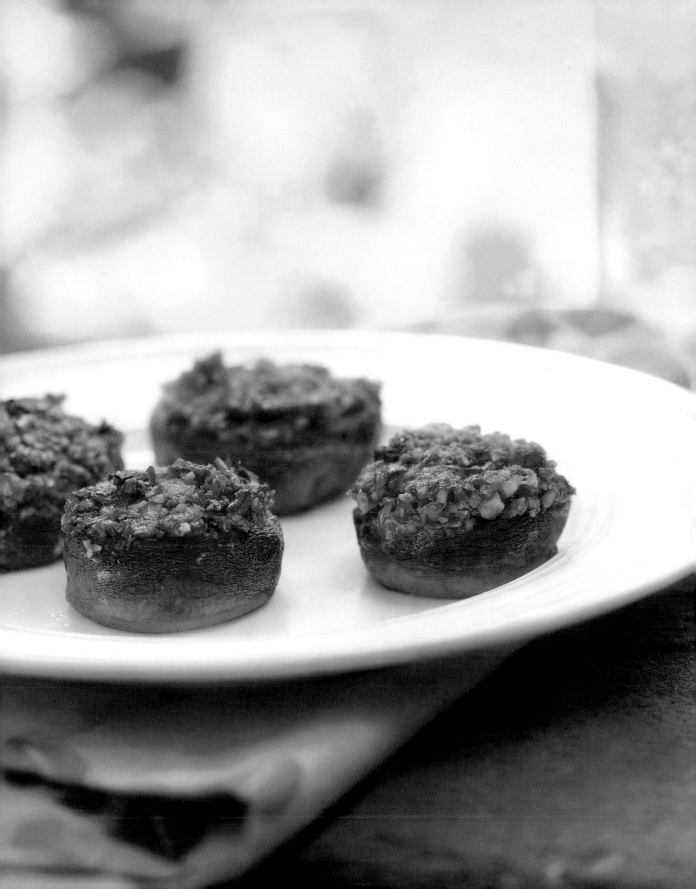

SEA VEGETABLES
Mineral-Rich Super Algae

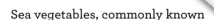

Sea vegetables, commonly known as seaweed, grow around the world and have a long history of use as food and medicine in Asian cultures. However, for myself the thought of seaweed conjures up childhood memories of Cape Cod vacations where ocean swimming inevitably meant getting tangled in masses of long, weedy strands that floated along the shoreline—not something I would have ever considered snacking on. But once I got my first taste of seaweed in my twenties—a simple seaweed and cucumber salad at an Asian restaurant in my Dupont Circle neighborhood—I was hooked. Packed with flavor and abundant in compounds that help support metabolism and weight, fight off cancer, and reduce risk factors associated with heart disease and diabetes, sea vegetables are ocean-to-plate superstars.

Iodine-Rich Algae Assists the Thyroid

Sea vegetables are a rich source of nutrients, including antioxidant vitamins A, C, and E and minerals like calcium, magnesium, and iron. They contain energy-boosting and stress-reducing B-complex vitamins, fiber, and omega-3 polyunsaturated fats, which help reduce inflammation and promote heart health. Seaweed is also one of the best natural sources of iodine, an essential trace element that helps support the thyroid, a gland that produces hormones involved in regulating metabolism, growth and development, mood, and body temperature. Although the iodine content of seaweed varies widely, ¼ ounce (about 7 g) of dried seaweed can contain as much as 4,500 micrograms of iodine—more than 2,250 to 4,500 percent of your daily needs.

Seaweed may also play a role in heart health and cancer prevention. Brown seaweed in particular contains important compounds called fucoidans, a class of sulfated polysaccharides (long chains of sulfur-containing sugars) with strong antioxidant, anti-inflammatory, anticancer, antiviral, and clot-preventing activities. Extracts of fucoidans from seaweed have been shown to reduce the growth and proliferation of certain cancer cells, and consuming sea vegetables rich in these compounds may help reduce the risk of skin, lung, breast, and other cancers. And while seaweed may help lower total and LDL ("bad") cholesterol levels, the blood-thinning effects of these compounds may also reduce the risk of clots associated with heart attack and stroke.

Fucoxanthins Support a Healthy Weight and Metabolism

Sea vegetables, particularly brown algae, contain metabolism-boosting and weight loss-promoting carotenoids called fucoxanthins. Researchers have found that these compounds stimulate proteins in the energy centers of fat cells involved in burning fat and boosting metabolism. In animal studies, extracts of fucoxanthin reduced both visceral fat (fat surrounding the organs) and the size of fat cells in obese mice, helping them to lose weight—in some cases by as much as 5 to 10 percent. These compounds also seem to help improve blood glucose levels and insulin resistance—important factors in diabetes. Human studies have shown similar results.

In a 2010 study, researchers found that obese women who consumed a supplement of fucoxanthin-containing brown seaweed extracts and pomegranate seed oil had significant reductions in body weight, body fat, liver fat, and waist circumference after sixteen weeks.

PUTTING IT INTO PRACTICE

Seaweed is classified into three main categories: green seaweed (*Chlorophycophyta*), which includes sea lettuce; brown seaweed (*Phaeophycophyta*), which includes kombu, wakame, and arame, and is often collectively referred to as kelp; and red seaweed (*Rhodophycophyta*), which includes nori, dulse, and agar agar. The flavor of seaweed varies among types, but tends to be quite salty with a mild to strong ocean flavor (some describe seaweed as having a somewhat fishy taste). And the texture of seaweed ranges from soft and chewy to hard and crisp, depending on the type and how it is prepared. You can find seaweed at most supermarkets and health food stores, where it is commonly available as a dry product that can be incorporated directly into recipes or rehydrated prior to consuming.

Nori, which is available as toasted or untoasted flat sheets, can be used to make sushi rolls. Small amounts of kombu can be added to soups for flavoring or cooked with beans to make them more digestible. Powdered or flaked dulse can be conveniently sprinkled on salads, soups, or other dishes for flavor and nutrition. And wakame, which can be rehydrated by soaking in water, makes a flavorful addition to soups, salads, and stir-fries. I generally recommend adding a serving or two of seaweed to your diet each week for a beneficial mineral boost. Some individuals enjoy seaweed more frequently, but because of its high sodium content—nearly 200 milligrams per ¼ cup (20 g)—salt-sensitive individuals may not be able to tolerate it more than once or twice a week.

CUCUMBER WAKAME SALAD

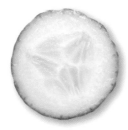

This nourishing salad combines mineral-rich wakame with hydrating cucumber and a sprinkle of calcium-friendly sesame seeds. Although the dressing is subtly spicy, I like to add a few extra pinches of cayenne pepper for an extra kick.

2 ounces (55 g) dried wakame flakes
1 medium-size cucumber
  Sea salt
1 tablespoon (8 g) sesame seeds
1 tablespoon (15 ml) rice vinegar
1 tablespoon (15 ml) sesame oil
1 tablespoon (20 g) agave syrup
  Several generous pinches of cayenne pepper

Yield: 4 servings

In a large bowl, cover the dried wakame flakes with cold water and soak for 4 to 6 minutes to rehydrate. Drain, rinse well, and pat dry.

Slice the cucumber paper thin (I use a mandolin) and place in a colander. Toss with a generous sprinkling of salt and let stand for 5 minutes. Rinse the cucumber slices to remove any salt, drain, and pat dry. Combine the wakame, cucumber, and sesame seeds in a mixing bowl.

In a separate bowl, whisk together the rice vinegar, sesame oil, agave syrup, and cayenne pepper. Drizzle the dressing lightly over the wakame and cucumber, toss to coat, and serve.

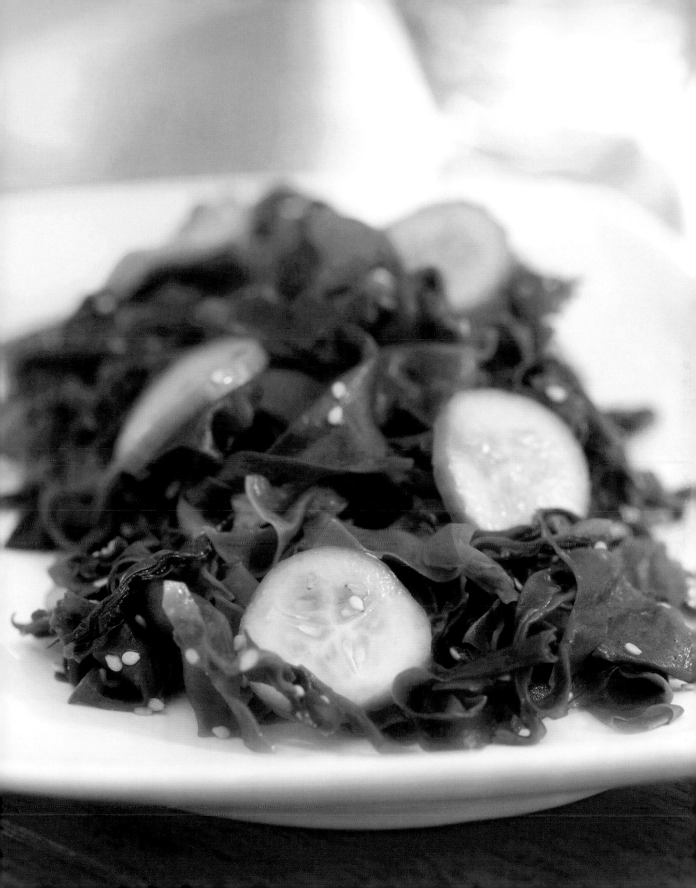

PUMPKIN
Cancer-Fighting Superfood

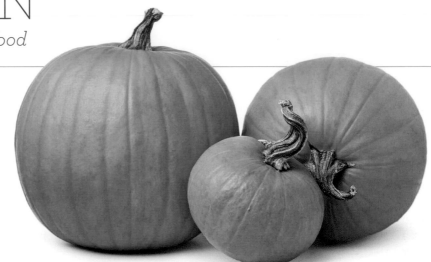

Growing up, I eagerly anticipated the arrival of October as my family and I would head to the nearest pumpkin patch or farm stand in search of perfectly sized and shaped pumpkins to carve and decorate for Halloween. I looked forward to making some pretty cool jack-o'-lanterns, but what I remember most was my dad's anticipation of all the pumpkin seeds we could eat. Together, we would scoop out piles and piles of the inner pulp and seeds from our pumpkins. We would sort them, rinse them, and lay them out on large cookie sheets to dry, and with a drizzle of oil and a sprinkle of salt, we would roast them in the oven. They made a great snack for the following week—or at least the following day (they didn't last long in our house).

Of course, the fall and early winter months also meant that my mom would be busy baking pumpkin pies, breads, and muffins, which we gladly devoured. Fortunately for us, pumpkins not only tasted good but gave our body a big boost of immune-supporting and cancer-fighting nutrients. So get ready to add this power food to your plate this fall for health and flavor.

Immune-Boosting Power of Vitamin A and Zinc

Pumpkins and other winter squash are often categorized as starchy vegetables, though technically they belong to the Cucurbitaceae family, which includes squash and melons. They are a perfect fall weather food, providing the nutrients needed to keep your body healthy and strong when the cool weather (and cold and flu season) sets in.

Pumpkins are a rich source of vitamins A, C, and E as well as minerals like potassium, magnesium, and calcium. One cup (245 g) of pureed pumpkin meets more than 700 percent of your daily vitamin A needs, and contains about 10 milligrams of vitamin C, an antioxidant that helps shorten the duration and severity of the common cold. Pumpkin seeds are an excellent source of zinc, a mineral that helps support the immune system and wound healing. A small serving of pumpkin seeds—about ¼ cup (16 g)—contains more than 2½ milligrams of zinc, 20 to 30 percent of your recommended daily allowance.

Heart-Healthy Phytosterols and Cancer-Crushing Carotenoids

Pumpkins are high in heart-healthy fiber (about 7 grams per cup [245 g] of pumpkin puree) and carotenoids like beta-, alpha-, and gamma-carotenes, which may protect against certain cancers, heart disease, and age-related diseases of the eye like macular degeneration and cataracts. Pumpkin seeds—and their oils—are also rich in phytosterols like beta-sitosterol, a compound that helps prevent the absorption of cholesterol and lowers both total and LDL ("bad") cholesterol levels.

In a study published in 2012, researchers found that treatment with pumpkin seed oil over a six-week period significantly reduced high blood pressure and normalized heart function in hypertensive rats. And the changes were similar to those treated with calcium channel blockers (drugs used to treat high blood pressure). More proof that food is medicine.

The carotenoids in pumpkin and the phytosterols in pumpkin seeds and oil may also play a role in cancer treatment and prevention. Studies have found that these compounds may reduce the risk of lung, colon, breast, prostate, and other cancers. In a study published in the *International Journal of Cancer*, researchers found that prostate cancer risk declined with increasing intakes of carotenoids (like alpha- and beta-carotene, lycopene, lutein, and zeaxanthin). And they found that the more carotenoid-rich foods (including pumpkin, spinach, tomatoes, and watermelon) men ate, the lower their risk of prostate cancer.

PUTTING IT INTO PRACTICE

Fresh pumpkins are in season from fall through early winter. You can store fresh pumpkins in a cool, dry place, where they will last for several months. To prepare a fresh pumpkin for cooking, simply remove the inner pulp and seeds and cut the pumpkin into chunks as you would any winter squash.

Pumpkins can be roasted or steamed and served as a side dish to accompany nearly any meal; I like to combine pumpkin with sautéed greens like chard and season with spices like cinnamon and nutmeg. You can also purée cooked pumpkin to create soups, sauces for pasta dishes, pie fillings, or mousses. Pumpkin seeds from fresh pumpkins can be rinsed, dried, and roasted for a protein-rich snack—or you can purchase raw, roasted, or sprouted pumpkin seeds, which can be tossed into trail mix, salads, and grain-based dishes. Pumpkin oil, which is the oil expressed from the seeds, can also be used to dress vegetable and grain-based salads.

PUMPKIN SPICE MILK

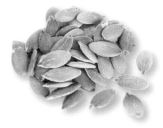

This creamy seed milk is packed with essential minerals, healthful fats, and phytonutrients. Sip it chilled or gently warmed—it's a great caffeine-free alternative to coffee and tea. It can also be stirred into bowls of oats, amaranth, or chia for extra flavor and nutrition.

1 cup (64 g) raw pumpkin seeds, soaked for 3 to 4 hours

4 cups (950 ml) filtered water

4 dates, pitted

2 tablespoons (28 g) coconut oil

1 teaspoon pure vanilla extract

1 teaspoon ground cinnamon

¼ teaspoon ground ginger

¼ teaspoon ground nutmeg

Pinch of sea salt

Yield: 2 servings

Drain and rinse the pumpkin seeds. Blend the seeds with the water in a high-speed blender for approximately 1 minute. Strain the milk into a separate pitcher using a nut milk bag or strainer. Rinse the blender container with water. Blend the strained milk with the remaining ingredients until smooth. Pour into tightly lidded glass jars and refrigerate. This milk is best served chilled or gently warmed. Shake well before serving.

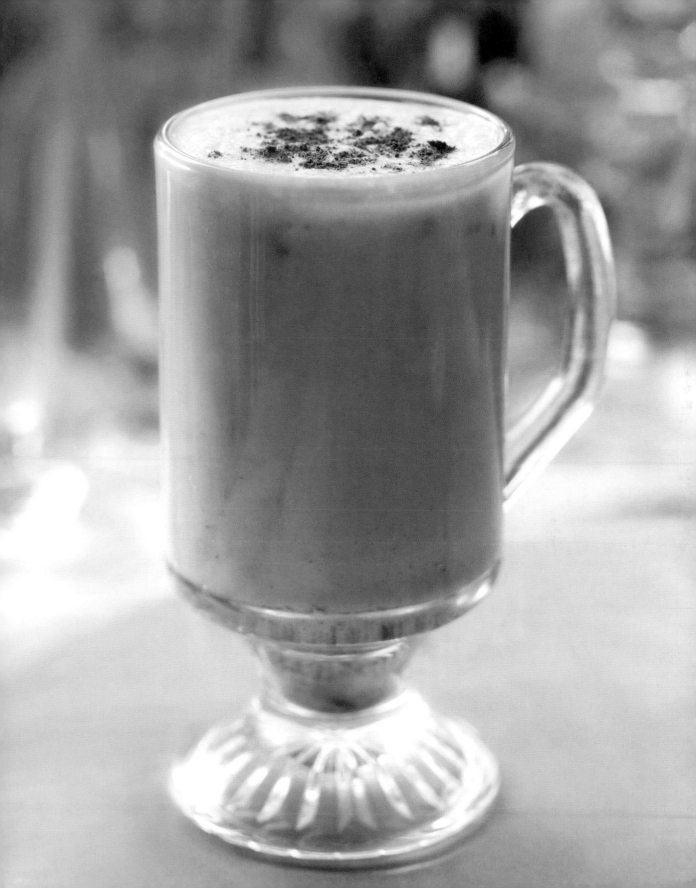

YACON
Prebiotic-Rich Super Root

SPOTLIGHT: PREBIOTICS AND PROBIOTICS

Probiotics are the beneficial bacteria (like *Lactobacilli* and *Bifidobacteria*) that are found in fermented foods or probiotic supplements. Prebiotics (like fructooligosaccharides [FOS]) are compounds that support the growth of these beneficial bacteria. In general, probiotics—and the prebiotics that "feed" them—may help improve digestion, boost the immune system, and enhance nutrient absorption. You can increase your intake of probiotics by consuming more fermented foods like sauerkraut, kimchi, miso, and kombucha. And you can boost your intake of prebiotics (like FOS and insulin) by eating more foods that contain them, such as yacon root, flax, greens, and berries.

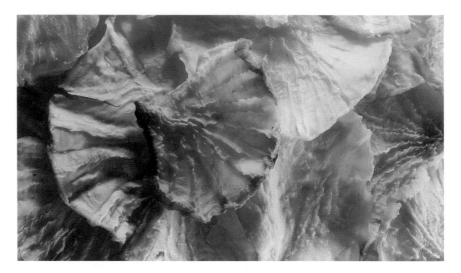

Yacon is a tuber (*Smallanthus sonchifolius*) native to the Andes Mountains in South America. *Yacón* means "water root," and indeed, it is a crisp and juicy water-rich vegetable (it can be eaten raw like a fruit) with the sweet flavor of an apple. But don't let the sweet taste of yacon fool you; this high-fiber vegetable may actually benefit those with high blood sugars. For centuries, Peruvians used yacon root—as well as its leaves—to treat high blood sugars and kidney problems. And researchers have found that its carbohydrates, which are in the form of fructooligosaccharides (FOS), cannot be absorbed by the body and therefore do not cause blood sugars to rise. For this reason, yacon is considered a wonderful alternative sweetener for those who are sensitive to sugar. And with beneficial FOS, antioxidants, and polyphenols that may improve digestion, lower blood fats, and even build strong bones, yacon is an emerging superfood for optimal health.

Super Root for a Healthy Gut

The FOS in yacon pass through the small and large intestines, where they are metabolized by the beneficial bacteria that reside there. FOS allows the "good" bacteria, like *Lactobacilli* and *Bifidobacteria*, to flourish, while crowding out the "bad" bacteria—and this provides some major benefits to us. Maintaining the right balance of bacteria in the gut helps improve digestion, boost immunity, and enhance nutrient absorption.

Researchers have found that FOS-rich yacon root may aid bowel function and prevent constipation by speeding up the time it takes for food to move through the colon. It may also help ease the symptoms of irritable bowel syndrome, diarrhea, and other digestive conditions, particularly when combined with a probiotic. Yacon root is also thought to inhibit the activity of cancer-causing compounds within the digestive tract.

In a study published in 2012, researchers found that when rats were fed dried extracts of yacon root—or a combination of yacon root and probiotic—they experienced a significant reduction in the numbers of aberrant crypt foci (ACF) in their colon. (ACF are abnormal, tubelike glands that are one of the first changes seen in the colon that may lead to colon cancer.)

PUTTING IT INTO PRACTICE

Yacon is cultivated around the world, and its peak season is in the fall when its tubers begin to develop. Once harvested, it can be stored in a cool, dry space, where it will keep for several months. During that time, its sweet flavor will actually intensify.

Fresh yacon can be peeled and eaten raw on its own or chopped and added to fruit or green salads (tossing it with lemon juice will prevent it from browning). A traditional South American fruit salad combines fresh yacon root with pineapple, mango, and papaya. Yacon can also be baked, roasted, or sautéed like other root vegetables.

Yacon syrup, dried yacon slices, and yacon powder are becoming more widely available at supermarkets and health food stores. Yacon syrup can be used as an alternative sweetener to honey, maple syrup, or agave syrup. You can drizzle it over pancakes, waffles, or a bowl of warm oats, or add it to smoothies and baked goods. Dried yacon slices are simply the sliced and dehydrated roots of yacon, which make a great snack alone. And yacon powder consists of sliced yacon roots that are dehydrated at low temperatures and ground into a fine powder. They can be used in baked goods as a substitute for other sweeteners—cup for cup or gram for gram—though the final flavor may vary slightly (researchers estimate that yacon has only 30 to 50 percent of the sweetness of regular sugar).

TROPICAL FRUIT SALAD

This simple fruit salad combines a few fresh tropical fruits with dried yacon root pieces and flaked coconut. I usually enjoy the natural sweetness of the fruits alone, but you can toss with a few squeezes of fresh orange juice or the creamy cashew dressing in this recipe.

- 1 small fresh pineapple, peeled and sliced (about 6 cups [990 g])
- 1 fresh mango, peeled and chopped (about 1 cup [175 g])
- 2 cups (340 g) sliced fresh strawberries
- 3 fresh kiwifruits, peeled and sliced (about 1 cup [178 g])
- ½ cup (70 g) raw cashews, soaked for 1 to 2 hours
- ¼ cup (80 g) agave syrup
- 1 tablespoon (15 ml) freshly squeezed lime juice
- ¼ cup (about 9 g) dried yacon root, torn or cut into bite-size pieces
- 2 tablespoons (10 g) unsweetened flaked coconut

Yield: 8 to 10 servings

Combine the pineapple, mango, strawberries, and kiwi in a large serving bowl. To make the dressing, drain and rinse the cashews. In a blender, combine the cashews with the agave syrup and lime juice and blend at high speed until thick and creamy. If the dressing is too thick, blend with a few extra squeezes of lime juice to thin. Pour the dressing over the fruit salad and stir to combine. Top with the dried yacon slices and coconut.

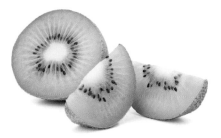

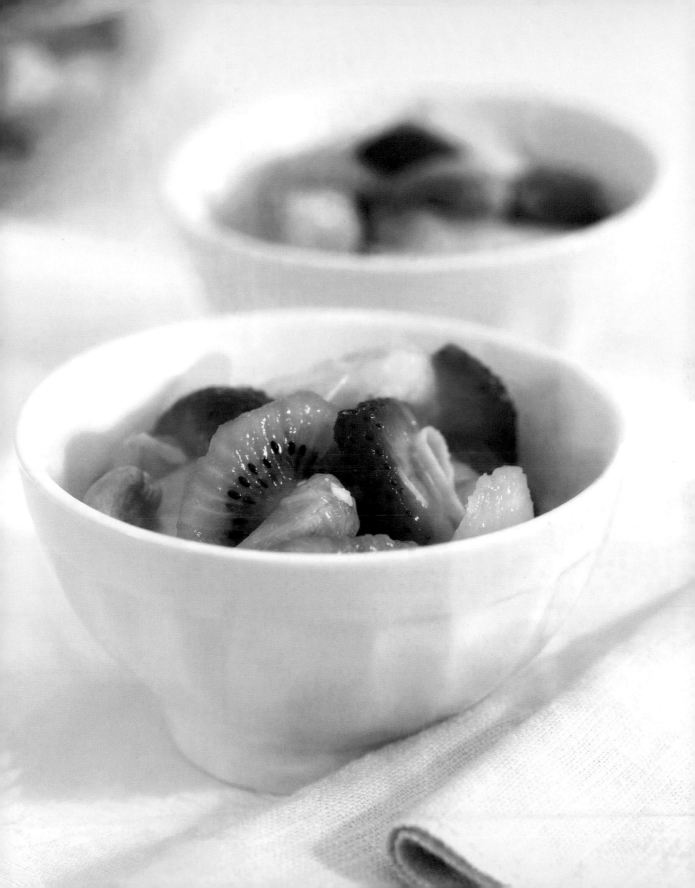

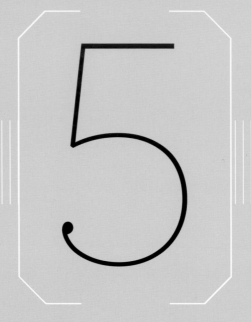

SUPER SEEDS
AND NUTS

*Chia Seeds, Flaxseeds, Hemp Seeds, Quinoa,
Sacha Inchi Seeds, Sesame Seeds, Walnuts*

These super nuts and seeds are the foods that help enhance strength and stamina. They provide a boost of easy-to-digest proteins to build and repair tissues and are packed with polyunsaturated omega-3 fatty acids that help fight inflammation. Add a handful or two of these nuts and seeds to your diet each day for good health.

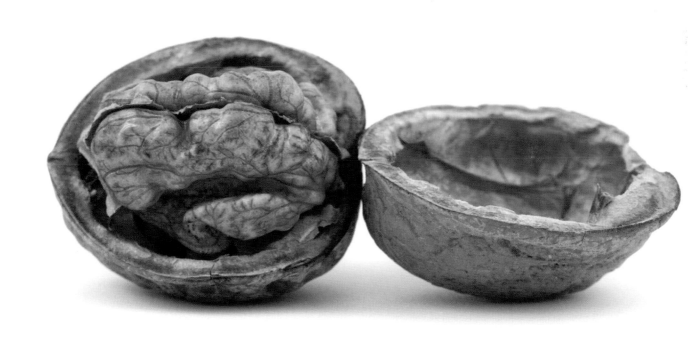

CHIA SEEDS

Super Seed for Sustained Energy

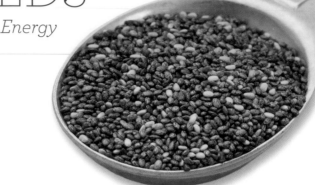

SPOTLIGHT: OMEGA-3 FATTY ACIDS

Omega-3 fatty acids are essential fats that your body cannot make, so they must be consumed from the foods you eat. These fatty acids include docosahexaenoic acid (DHA), eicosapentaenoic acid (EPA), and alpha-linolenic acid (ALA), the latter of which is found in plant foods and converted to DHA and EPA in the body. Omega-3 fatty acids help reduce inflammation and are associated with lower blood cholesterol and triglyceride levels, reduced risk of heart disease and depression, and protection against neurological diseases like Alzheimer's disease and dementia. You can boost your intake of plant-based omega-3 fatty acids by adding chia, flax, hemp, and walnuts to your diet.

Chia seeds are the edible seeds of a desert plant (*Salvia hispanica*) native to Mexico and the southwestern United States. The Mayan word for "strength," chia was a dietary staple of the Mayans and Aztecs, who used it to increase strength, energy, and stamina. Even today it is often referred to as "runner's food." Indeed, chia is a concentrated source of energy-producing carbohydrates and numerous vitamins, minerals, antioxidants, and inflammation-fighting fatty acids. With an impressive array of health-promoting compounds— all packed into tiny black and white seeds that are incredibly simple to work with—chia is becoming a dietary staple in the modern food world.

Calcium-Rich Chia Builds a Strong Body

Chia seeds are an excellent source of energy, with about 12 grams of carbohydrate and nearly 5 grams of protein packed into a single ounce (28 g). They are also a good source of minerals, including blood-building iron, stress-relieving magnesium, and bone-building calcium. In fact, a 1-ounce (28 g) serving of dried chia seeds boasts a striking 179 milligrams of calcium—nearly 20 percent of the average adult's daily needs—and more than the amount in a ½-cup (120 ml) serving of milk. And although a mere ounce of these little seeds contains more than 8 grams of fat, more than 80 percent of that fat is in the form of heart-healthy polyunsaturated omega-3 fatty acids, like alpha-linolenic acid.

In addition to its healthful fats, chia is also an incredibly good source of dietary fiber. It contains about 10 grams of fiber per ounce (28 g)—30 to 40 percent of your daily needs. And because these little fiber-rich seeds also have the unique ability to expand when added to water, some experts believe that in the stomach, they may slow the digestion and release of sugar into the bloodstream, benefiting those looking to lose weight and control blood sugars.

Fiber May Benefit Blood Sugars

Chia seeds may help improve blood sugars and risk factors associated with heart disease. Some animal studies have shown that chia-enriched diets may improve insulin resistance, normalize blood lipids, and even reduce the accumulation of visceral fat (the fat surrounding the organs) in the body. In a study published in 2012, researchers found that rats whose high-fat, high-carbohydrate diets were supplemented with 5 percent chia seeds over an eight-week period had improved insulin sensitivity and glucose tolerance, decreased abdominal and liver fat, and reduced inflammation in both the heart and liver compared to the control group. Similar results have been seen in humans.

In a study published in 2007 in *Diabetes Care,* researchers found that adding about 37 grams (approximately 2½ tablespoons) of chia to the diets of adults with type 2 diabetes reduced systolic blood pressure and markers of inflammation compared to the control group. And in a small study published in the *European Journal of Clinical Nutrition* in 2010, researchers found that adults who consumed a chia-enriched bread—which contained varying amounts of chia up to 24 grams (approximately 2 tablespoons)—had dose-dependent reductions in blood sugar levels after eating (meaning that the more chia baked into the bread, the greater the effect.).

PUTTING IT INTO PRACTICE

Chia seeds can be found in most supermarkets or health food stores. Try adding an ounce (28 g) or two of whole chia seeds to salads, smoothies, and hot and cold cereals for a boost of fiber, protein, healthy fat, and calcium. Unlike flaxseeds, the nutrients in chia seeds can be absorbed by your body without grinding them. However, chia seeds can also be ground into flour for baking, and because they absorb liquids, they are a great thickening agent for sauces, soups, smoothies, dressings, and puddings—without altering the taste as they have no distinct flavor of their own. In fact, you can make your own chia pudding by combining whole chia seeds and your favorite nondairy milk: Simply add 2 tablespoons (28 g) of whole chia seeds to ½ cup (120 ml) of liquid and refrigerate overnight. Once the pudding is formed, you can experiment with the flavor and texture by adding your own selection of fresh or dried fruit, nuts, and spices. Simple and nutritious!

POMEGRANATE-GREEN TEA CHIA PUDDING

I love sipping on iced green tea with a splash of pomegranate juice, and this thick and creamy chia pudding combines those two antioxidant-rich superstars into one bowl. Whether you soak this dish overnight or assemble it first thing in the morning, it provides a simple and nutritious start to your day.

½ cup (120 ml) unsweetened almond milk

½ cup (120 ml) pomegranate juice

1 tablespoon (20 g) agave syrup

1 teaspoon matcha green tea powder

½ teaspoon pure vanilla extract

¼ cup (56 g) white or black chia seeds

¼ cup (44 g) pomegranate arils

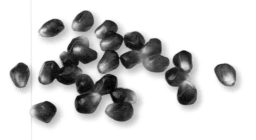

Yield: 1 to 2 servings

For same-day preparation: In a small bowl, whisk together the almond milk, pomegranate juice, agave syrup, matcha tea, and vanilla extract. Add the chia seeds and stir thoroughly to combine. Allow the mixture to rest for 30 minutes, stirring every 5 to 10 minutes until thick. Pour into a serving bowl, top with the pomegranate arils, and serve.

For overnight soaking: Combine all the ingredients, except for the pomegranate arils. Transfer the chia pudding mixture to a tightly lidded glass jar (I like to use Ball mason jars), shake, and refrigerate. If you are not heading straight to bed, give the pudding a shake every 5 to 10 minutes until bedtime. In the morning, give the pudding a final shake or stir, pour into a serving bowl, top with the pomegranate arils, and serve.

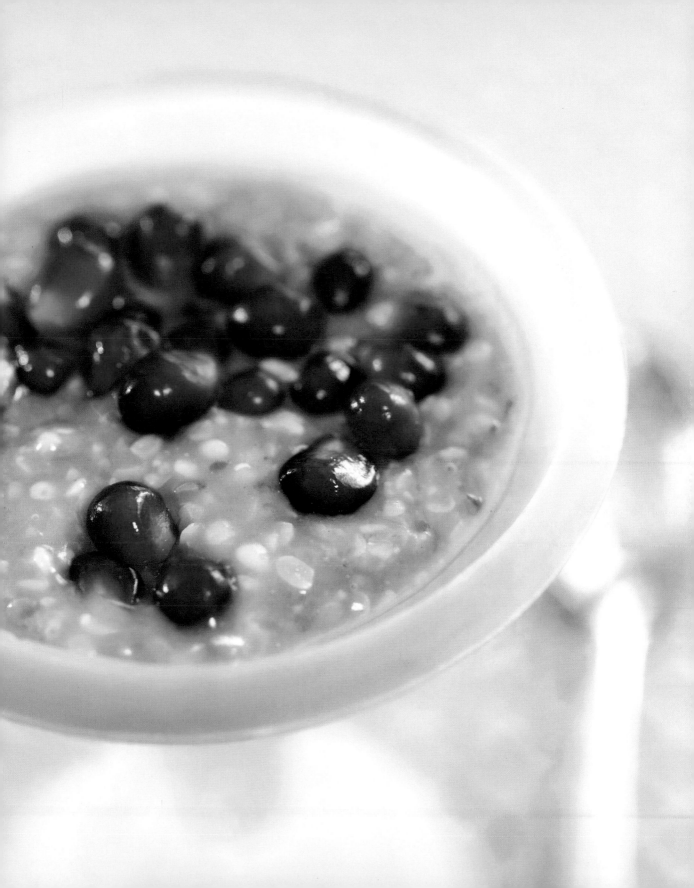

FLAXSEEDS
Lignan-Rich Super Seed

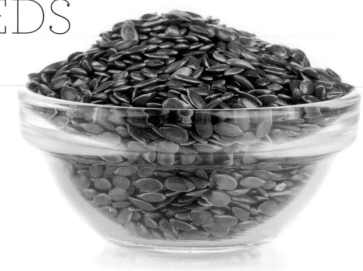

**SUPERFOOD KITCHEN TIP:
FLAXSEED EGG REPLACER**

Flaxseeds can be used in most baked dishes as an egg replacer. For each egg, simply mix 1 tablespoon (7 g) of ground flaxseed meal with 3 tablespoons (45 ml) of water. Let stand at room temperature for a minute or two until the mixture becomes gel-like. Add the flax and water mixture to your recipe just as you would an egg. So easy—and good for you!

Flaxseeds, also known as linseeds, are the tiny seeds of the *Linum usitatissimum* plant. They are an excellent source of heart-healthy fiber and essential omega-3 fatty acids. They are also the richest known source of cancer-fighting phytochemicals called lignans—far surpassing that of any other plant food. From lowering cholesterol to reducing the risk of heart disease and certain cancers, flaxseed is a powerful superfood for good health—and one that is super simple to add to your daily diet.

Flaxseeds Full of Fiber and Omega-3 Fatty Acids

Just 2 tablespoons (24 g) of whole flaxseeds supply about 6 grams of dietary fiber—nearly a quarter of your daily needs. They are also a good source of calcium, with over 400 milligrams per cup (168 g)—more than an equivalent serving of milk. And although flaxseeds are a rich source of fat—3 to 4 grams per tablespoon (12 g)—more than half of that fat is in the form of heart-healthy alpha-linolenic acid (ALA), an inflammation-fighting omega-3 fatty acid.

Heart-Healthy, Cancer-Fighting Super Seed

Fiber- and ALA-rich flaxseeds are good for the heart and have been associated with a reduced risk of atherosclerosis (hardening of the arteries) and heart disease. Flaxseeds may help lower total and LDL ("bad") cholesterol levels, reduce blood pressure, and make platelets (the blood cells involved in clotting) less sticky and less likely to cause the clots that can lead to heart attack and stroke. A few studies have found that these tiny seeds may also help lower blood sugars and hemoglobin A1c (a marker of long-term blood sugar control) in individuals with type 2 diabetes.

Flaxseeds are also an excellent source of lignans, polyphenols with strong anti-inflammatory and antioxidant properties. Often classified as phytoestrogens (weak plant estrogens that compete with

152 | POWERFUL PLANT-BASED SUPERFOODS

the body's natural estrogens during certain chemical reactions), lignans may help slow the growth of certain estrogen-driven cancers, such as breast cancer, as well as other cancers including those of the colon, prostate, and lungs. In addition to flaxseeds, other good sources of lignans include sesame, pumpkin, and sunflower seeds; whole grains; beans; berries; and nuts.

PUTTING IT INTO PRACTICE

Flaxseeds are available in most supermarkets and health food stores. I recommend buying either whole flaxseeds or ground flaxseed meal and storing in a tightly lidded container in the refrigerator or freezer. If you purchase whole flaxseeds, grind them before eating to make the beneficial nutrients—including the healthy fats and lignans—more readily available for digestion and absorption. You can grind whole flaxseeds using a small coffee grinder or purchase ground flaxseeds (sometimes called milled flaxseed or flaxseed meal) in bulk or bags. Although the beneficial fats and phytonutrients in whole flaxseeds cannot be absorbed without grinding, whole flaxseeds are still a great addition to the diet for those simply looking to increase fiber intake.

A tablespoon (7 g) or two of ground flaxseed meal makes an excellent addition to salads, soups, and smoothies. It can also be incorporated into baked goods as an added source of nutrients or as an egg replacer. Whole flaxseeds can be sprinkled onto cereals or baked into breads. Many research studies have found that upward of 40 to 50 grams of flaxseeds (3 to 4 tablespoons) may offer such benefits as reducing the incidence of hot flashes or lowering cholesterol levels. However, because flax is so high in fiber, some individuals may experience upset stomach and bloating when consuming these amounts. As with any high-fiber food, start by adding small amounts—around a teaspoon or two—and gradually increase your intake. And be sure to drink plenty of water. Increasing fiber intake without increasing fluid intake can also contribute to constipation and bloating.

CHOCOLATE CHIP
FLAX COOKIES

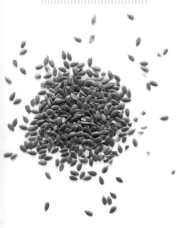

Flax is a great addition—both for health and its binding properties—to this modified version of the traditional chocolate chip cookie I grew up on. I use an all-purpose, gluten-free flour in this recipe (Bob's Red Mill Gluten-Free All Purpose Flour is my favorite), but if you don't have celiac disease, gluten intolerance, or a wheat allergy, feel free to use an equivalent amount of regular whole wheat or whole wheat pastry flour.

1 tablespoon (7 g) ground flaxseed meal

3 tablespoons (45 ml) water

1 cup (136 g) all-purpose, gluten-free flour

½ teaspoon baking soda

½ teaspoon sea salt

½ cup (113 g) coconut oil, liquefied

½ cup (96 g) cane sugar

¼ cup (48 g) brown sugar

½ teaspoon pure vanilla extract

1 cup (170 g) dark chocolate chips

½ cup (60 g) walnuts, chopped (optional)

Yield: about 2 dozen cookies

Preheat the oven to 375°F (190°C, or gas mark 5). Line two cookie sheets with parchment paper.

In a small bowl, stir together the flaxseed meal and water. Set aside for a few minutes to thicken.

Combine the flour, baking soda, and salt and set aside. In a separate bowl, beat together the coconut oil, sugars, vanilla, and flaxseed mixture at medium speed. Gradually beat in the dry mixture at low speed until a ball of cookie dough forms. Fold in the chocolate chips and walnuts (if using) and drop by tablespoons (15 g mounds) onto the prepared cookie sheets.

Bake for 8 to 10 minutes until lightly browned. Remove from the oven, let cool on the cookie sheets for 1 to 2 minutes, and then transfer to cooling racks.

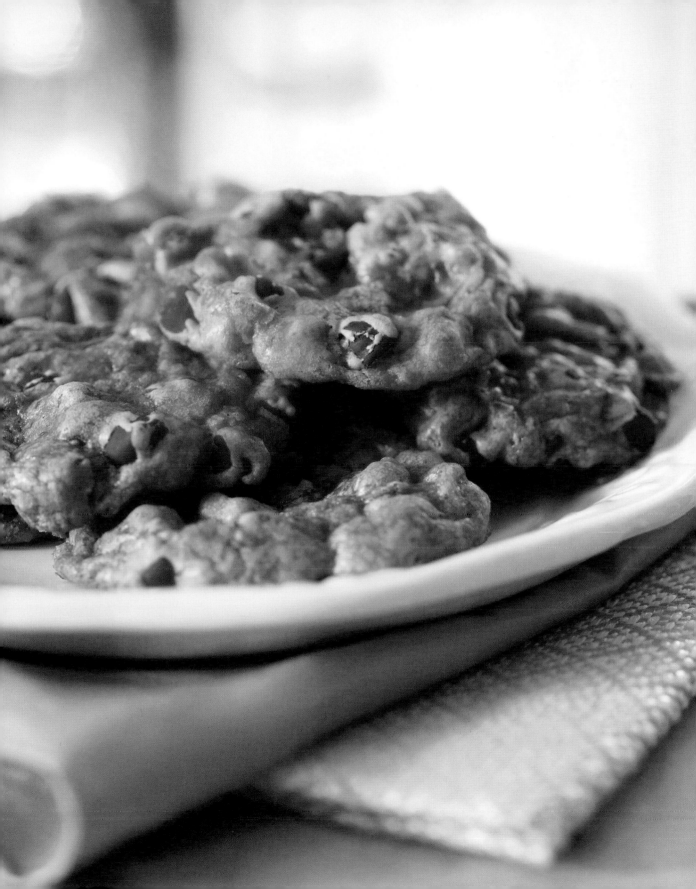

HEMP SEEDS
Protein- and Fat-Rich Super Seed

SPOTLIGHT: OMEGA-3 AND OMEGA-6 FATTY ACIDS

Both omega-3 and omega-6 fatty acids are important to your health—you just need to consume them in the right balance. Experts estimate that the ideal ratio for consumption of omega-6 to omega-3 fatty acids is 1:1. However, most Americans consume these fats in a 10:1 ratio, which means we are consuming way too many omega-6 fatty acids. Not that these fats aren't important to your diet, but when you consume too many of them—typically in the form of vegetable oils from processed foods—inflammation occurs. To improve your balance of omega fatty acids, the remedy is simple: reduce the amount of processed foods you eat and increase your intake of omega-3 fats with foods like walnuts, hemp, chia, and flax.

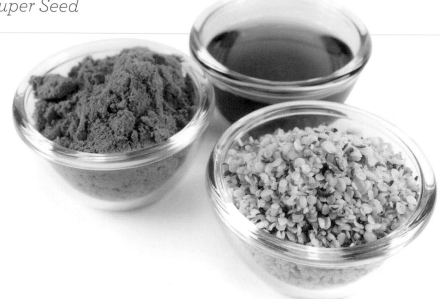

I've worked with athletes on and off for more than fifteen years, and I am always in search of the best nutrient-dense whole foods to both support their intense training and protect their bodies from the stressful effects of such training. Fortunately, hemp seeds are one of those nutrient-dense whole foods. An easy-to-digest protein, hemp seeds are also rich in inflammation-fighting essential fats, which make them an optimal choice for athletes and nonathletes alike.

The Incredible Protein-Packed Hemp Seed

Hemp seeds come from an industrialized, nondrug type of annual herbaceous plant (*Cannibis sativa*). They are an excellent source of easy-to-digest protein that include all nine essential amino acids in levels that are close to those of the complete proteins found in animal products and soy. They are also a significant source of arginine, a nonessential amino acid that appears to benefit the heart. Found in protein-rich foods, including plant foods like soy and nuts, arginine helps keep the blood vessels functioning optimally.

When it comes to the quantity of protein and other nutrients in hemp seeds, don't let the size of this little seed fool you. A single ounce (28 g) of shelled hemp seeds contains about 7 grams of easy-to-digest protein (slightly more than one large egg), 10 grams of heart-healthy fats, and nearly 8 grams of dietary fiber. Hemp is also a good source of vitamins like the antioxidant vitamin E and minerals like potassium, magnesium, and iron, to name a few. In fact, just 2 tablespoons (15 grams) of hemp powder meets more than a quarter of your daily iron needs.

Beautiful Balance of Omega-3 and Omega-6 Fatty Acids

Hemp seeds are high in omega-3 and omega-6 fatty acids, and together these fats may help reduce the risk of diseases affected by inflammation, including heart disease, cancer, diabetes, and autoimmune diseases like rheumatoid arthritis. They also have a protective effect on the brain and skin.

Omega-3 fatty acids are especially known for their potent inflammation-fighting effects. But although omega-6 fatty acids—the ones found in some vegetable oils, nuts, and seeds—don't tend to receive quite the same fanfare as the omega-3 fatty acids, they are still important to our health, especially our heart. Hemp seeds are an excellent source of linoleic acid, an omega-6 fatty acid that may help lower total and LDL ("bad") cholesterol and triglyceride levels, maintain healthy blood pressure, and prevent the formation of clots associated with heart attack and stroke. Together, these fats help fight inflammation in the body and reduce the risk of certain chronic diseases.

PUTTING IT INTO PRACTICE

Hemp can be purchased in the form of raw, shelled seeds, hemp seed powder, and hemp seed oil. The seeds have a mild, nutty flavor and are excellent additions to salads—simply toss a tablespoon (8 g) or two into your salad for a boost of healthy protein and fat. Hemp powder or flour is made of finely milled seeds that can be used in smoothies and shakes or as flour for baking. Adding 2 to 3 tablespoons (15 to 23 g) of powder will give you an additional 10 to 16 grams of high-quality, easy-to-digest protein. Hempseed oil is a cold-pressed oil that is green in color and best used as a dressing for salads and other cold dishes; mix a few tablespoons (about 45 ml) with squeeze of lemon juice and toss with your favorite veggies, greens, or grains to enhance your intake of beneficial fatty acids.

NO-BAKE CHOCOLATE BERRY HEMP BITES

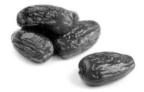

The natural sugars in dates combined with high-protein hemp seeds, nuts, and berries to make these no-bake bites the ultimate energy snack. They are sweet and chewy—with an added crunch from antioxidant-rich cacao nibs. Enjoy at home or on the go.

1½ cups (267 g) pitted dates
1 cup (145 g) raw almonds
½ cup (60 g) hemp seeds, divided
½ cup (56 g) dried goji berries
¼ cup (32 g) raw cacao nibs
2 tablespoons (40 g) agave syrup

Yield: 50 bites

Combine all the ingredients (except ¼ cup [30 g] of the hemp seeds, for rolling) in a food processor and pulse into a coarse and slightly sticky meal. The mixture should stick together when pressed with the fingertips. If the mixture appears too dry, add one to two more dates or a squirt of agave syrup and process. If the mixture is too sticky, add a few almonds and process. Roll the mixture into teaspoon-size balls and dredge in hemp seeds to coat.

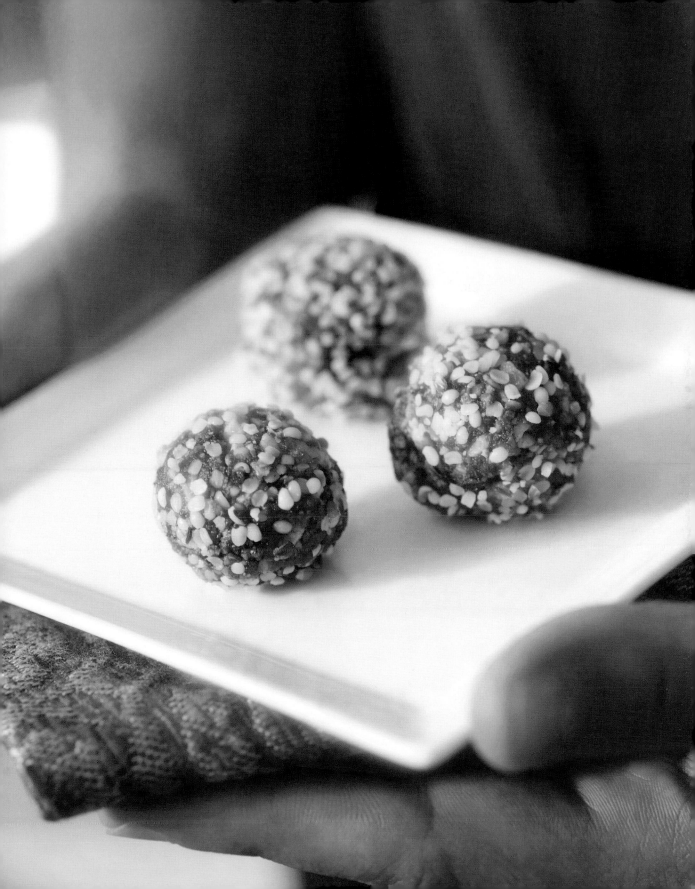

QUINOA
Complete Protein Super Seed

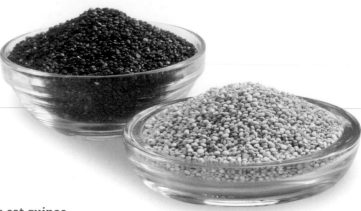

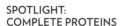

Quinoa is a complete protein that contains adequate levels of all nine essential amino acids. Nutrition experts—myself included—once thought that high-quality, complete proteins came only from animal products. How wrong we were! Researchers have classified the protein of several plant foods—like quinoa, soy (including edamame, tofu, tempeh, and miso), and possibly the emerging sacha inchi seeds—as complete proteins. Of course, almost all foods contain some protein, and you can easily meet your protein needs by eating a variety of plant foods—both complete and incomplete sources of protein—over the course of each day (no special combining needed!).

When you eat quinoa
(*Chenopodium quinoa*), you are eating the super seeds of an Amaranthacean plant that is related to beets, spinach, chard, and amaranth. This superfood is often classified as a grain (after all, it is cooked, prepared, and consumed similar to traditional grains), but is technically a seed—and one that has a long history of use as food and medicine. Native to South America, quinoa has been cultivated along the Andes Mountains for more than five thousand years. The Incans often referred to it as the "mother grain" and consumed it for strength and stamina. Today, quinoa is growing in popularity and enjoyed for both its taste and nutritional properties. Not only is it the least allergenic of all grains (it is naturally gluten free), but this pseudograin, as it is sometimes called, also seems to have a greater nutritional value than traditional grains. Quinoa is packed with amino acids, minerals, vitamins, and antioxidants that may help reduce the risk factors associated with diabetes and heart disease, boost brain function, and ease anxiety.

Protein- and Mineral-Rich Seed May Ease Stress
Quinoa is probably best known for its unique content of high-quality, easy-to-digest protein. One cup (185 g) of cooked quinoa has about 8 grams of complete protein (more than an egg), which includes adequate levels of all nine essential amino acids—and a similar amino acid profile to casein, a milk protein. It also contains higher levels of the amino acids cysteine, methionine, and lysine than do most plant foods. Additionally, quinoa contains substantial amounts of tryptophan, an essential amino acid that is involved in mood, sleep, and the production of serotonin (a "feel-good" chemical in the body).

Quinoa is also packed with minerals like calcium, magnesium, iron, copper, and zinc—and in amounts higher than most other grains. One cup (185 g) of cooked quinoa contains nearly 120 milligrams of magnesium—30 to 40 percent of your daily needs. Often referred to as a calming mineral, magnesium helps relax blood vessels and muscles (including the heart), may reduce the risk of high blood pressure and stroke, and may even benefit those suffering from migraines. It may also help reduce stress and improve sleep. In one animal study, researchers found that quinoa helped protect brain cells, reduce anxiety, and improve memory in stressed rats—and they attribute the beneficial effects to the combination of quinoa's vitamins, minerals, and amino acids.

Low-Glycemic-Index Ideal for Those with Diabetes

Quinoa may help lower risk factors associated with diabetes and heart disease—and even promote a healthy weight. A low-glycemic-index super seed (it won't cause a sharp rise in blood sugars when consumed), quinoa is rich in heart-healthy, polyunsaturated omega-3 fatty acids; antioxidant vitamins A, C, and E; and polyphenols like iso-flavones (plant estrogens that may help build strong bones, promote heart health, and reduce the risk of certain cancers). It is also a rich source of dietary fiber; 1 cup (185 g) of cooked quinoa contains about 5 grams of fiber—15 to 20 percent of your daily needs.

Not surprisingly, researchers have found that quinoa may have antiobesity, antidiabetes, and lipid-lowering effects. In animal studies, rats given extracts of quinoa have experienced weight and fat losses, as well as prevention of weight or fat gains, when fed high-fat or high-sugar diets. They have also shown improvements in blood sugar and insulin levels and in some cases, reductions in triglyceride and total and LDL ("bad") cholesterol levels. In a study published in *Plant Foods for Human Nutrition* in 2010, researchers noted significant reductions in total and LDL cholesterol, triglyceride, and glucose levels in rats whose "normal" or high-fructose diets were supplemented with quinoa. And while they found that quinoa-enriched diets did not increase HDL ("good") cholesterol levels, these diets did prevent fructose-induced decreases in HDL.

PUTTING IT INTO PRACTICE

Quinoa is widely available at supermarkets and health food stores, where you are likely to find it in the bulk or gluten-free departments. Store quinoa in tightly lidded containers in a cool, dry place, where it will last for several months.

When cooked, quinoa becomes light and fluffy with a slight crunch and mildly nutty flavor. You should always rinse quinoa thoroughly before cooking to remove the bitter saponins that coat the outside of the seed. Quinoa can be cooked on the stovetop: In a saucepan, combine 1 cup (173 g) of raw quinoa with 2 cups (475 ml) of water or vegetable stock, bring it to a boil, cover, reduce the heat, and allow it to simmer until done, about 15 minutes.

Alternatively, you can toast quinoa before cooking to bring out its nutty flavor: after rinsing, dry-roast it in a pan on the stovetop for 3 to 5 minutes. And if you prefer to consume quinoa uncooked, you can sprout it: after rinsing, simply soak it in water for 24 hours, drain, rinse, and serve—topped with your favorite vegetables, nuts, seeds, and herbs and spices.

Quinoa is a great alternative to most other traditional cereals and grains. Toss it into green salads for a protein boost or mix it with beans, seeds, and vegetables for a nutrient-packed main meal. It also makes a great breakfast cereal. Combine quinoa with fresh or dried fruits, nuts, spices like cinnamon, and a drizzle of maple or agave syrup for a stellar morning treat.

SPRING QUINOA SALAD

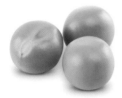

This spring salad is a simple mixture of two of my favorite spring foods: fresh peas and garlic scapes (the edible tops of garlic plants). There is really no substitute for garlic scapes in terms of flavor, but if you don't have them on hand, you can simply toss in an equivalent amount of raw scallions for a little boost of flavor and added crunch.

1½ cups (260 g) raw quinoa

3 cups (700 ml) water

Sea salt

¼ cup (60 ml) plus 1 teaspoon extra-virgin olive oil, divided

½ cup (50 g) garlic scapes, chopped

2 cups (300 g) fresh or frozen peas (thaw if frozen)

2 tablespoons (28 ml) freshly squeezed lemon juice

1 teaspoon agave syrup

1 teaspoon Dijon mustard

1 clove garlic, crushed

1 teaspoon chopped fresh flat-leaf parsley

1 teaspoon chopped fresh basil

Freshly ground pepper

Yield: 6 to 8 servings

Rinse the quinoa in a strainer. Place the quinoa, water, and a pinch of sea salt in a medium-size pot and bring to a boil. Cover, reduce the heat, and simmer until the water is absorbed, about 20 minutes. Remove from the heat, fluff with a fork, and transfer to a serving bowl.

Heat 1 teaspoon of the olive oil in a small skillet over medium heat. Add the chopped garlic scapes and sauté until soft, about 5 minutes. Add the scapes to the serving bowl containing the quinoa. Stir in the peas and set aside.

In a small bowl, whisk together the remaining ¼ cup (60 ml) of olive oil and the lemon juice, agave syrup, Dijon mustard, garlic, parsley, and basil. Season with salt and freshly ground pepper to taste. Pour the dressing over the quinoa and stir to combine. You can serve this dish warm, at room temperature, or chilled.

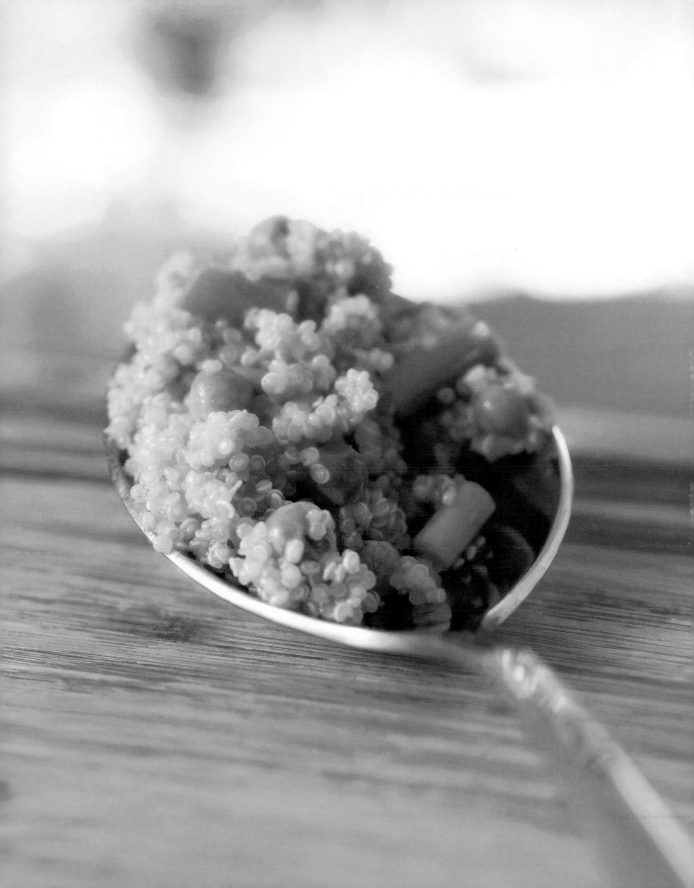

SACHA INCHI SEEDS
New Seed on the Block

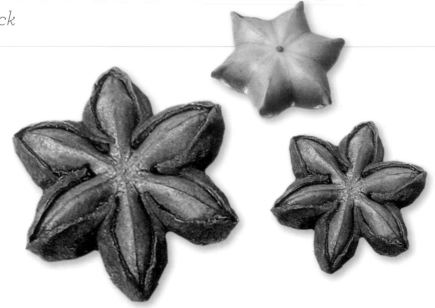

Vitamin E is an antioxidant that protects your cells from the damaging effects of free radicals. It also aids the immune system and acts as a natural vasodilator (it helps relax the blood vessels). A tablespoon (15 ml) of sacha inchi seed oil meets about 120 percent of your daily vitamin E needs (in addition to containing cancer-fighting carotenoids—like beta-carotene—and more than a dozen heart-healthy polyphenols). Other good sources of vitamin C include almonds, sunflower seeds, and hazel-nuts, and small amounts can even be found in green vegetables like spinach and broccoli.

Sacha inchi seeds are the edible seeds of star-shaped green fruits from a plant (*Plukenetia volubilis*) native to South America. Growing in the Andes, sacha inchi seeds have been consumed for thousands of years. However, these emerging super seeds, also known as Inca peanuts, are newbies in the world of superfoods. There is limited research on sacha inchi seeds, but as researchers begin to learn more about their nutrient composition, it is clear that they may confer some of the health benefits seen in similarly structured superfoods.

Sacha inchi seeds are rich in easy-to-digest proteins, contain a nice blend of essential fatty acids, and are a good source of antioxidant vitamins, minerals, and phytochemicals that put them right up there with more established super seeds like hemp, chia, and flax.

Protein Powerhouse

A single ounce (28 g) of sacha inchi seeds boasts an impressive 8 to 9 grams of easy-to-digest protein—more than you would find in a single egg. And according to researchers at Florida State University, sacha inchi seeds appear to be a complete source of protein, meaning that they not only contain all nine essential amino acids, but do so in levels and patterns deemed adequate by the World Health Organization and the Food and Agricultural Organization of the United Nations.

In addition, an ounce (28 g) of the seeds or a tablespoon (15 ml) of sacha inchi seed oil contains about 14 grams of fat—and an estimated 90 percent of that fat is in the form of heart-healthy unsaturated fats, which we know may help lower cholesterol levels (especially when they replace saturated fats in the diet). Researchers have found that about half of those unsaturated fats are in the form of anti-inflammatory omega-3 fatty acids like alpha-linolenic acid, while about 35 percent are in the form of omega-6 fatty acids like linoleic acid. And contrary to popular belief, small amounts of these omega-6 fats are important for good health.

Although excess amounts of omega-6 fatty acids—which most people consume in the form of vegetable oils from processed foods—can actually cause inflammation, the ratio of omega-3 and omega-6 fats in sacha inchi seeds appears to be ideal for supporting good health without promoting inflammation.

PUTTING IT INTO PRACTICE

As sacha inchi seeds continue to grow in popularity, they are becoming more widely available at supermarkets and health food stores. As of this writing, my local natural food store had just begun carrying the seeds. Whole sacha inchi seeds are roasted (according to one manufacturer I spoke with, they cannot be digested in their raw form because of a toxic protein they contain) and can be enjoyed alone as a snack or tossed into salads, trail mix, or homemade energy bars. A 1-ounce (28 g) serving—a small handful—will give you a nice boost of beneficial fats, protein, and around 5 grams of dietary fiber (about 20 percent of your daily needs). Sacha inchi oil, which is pressed from the seeds, has a light, nutty flavor and makes a great alternative to olive or hemp oils in salad dressings. Use sacha inchi oil with your favorite vinegar or freshly squeezed lemon juice in a 3:1 ratio and season with fresh herbs, dried spices, and a little freshly ground salt and pepper.

GINGERY BEET AND CARROT SALAD

One of my favorite juice combinations—especially in the fall—is sweet carrot, beet, and ginger juice. Grated beets and carrots combine in this recipe with a ginger-based dressing that incorporates the nutty flavor of sacha inchi oil. You can enjoy this dish alone or toss on top of a leafy green salad for added flavor and color. I also like the crunch of a few toasted sacha inchi seeds sprinkled on top.

2 cups (240 g) peeled and grated raw beets

2 cups (220 g) peeled and grated raw carrots

3 tablespoons (45 ml) extra-virgin sacha inchi seed oil

1 tablespoon (15 ml) raw apple cider vinegar

1 teaspoon grated fresh ginger

1 teaspoon agave syrup

Pinch of sea salt

¼ cup (42 g) roasted sacha inchi seeds, chopped

Yield: 4 servings

Combine the beets and carrots in a small serving bowl. Whisk together the oil, vinegar, ginger, agave syrup, and salt. Pour the vinaigrette over the salad and toss to coat. Top with the chopped sacha inchi seeds and serve.

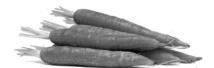

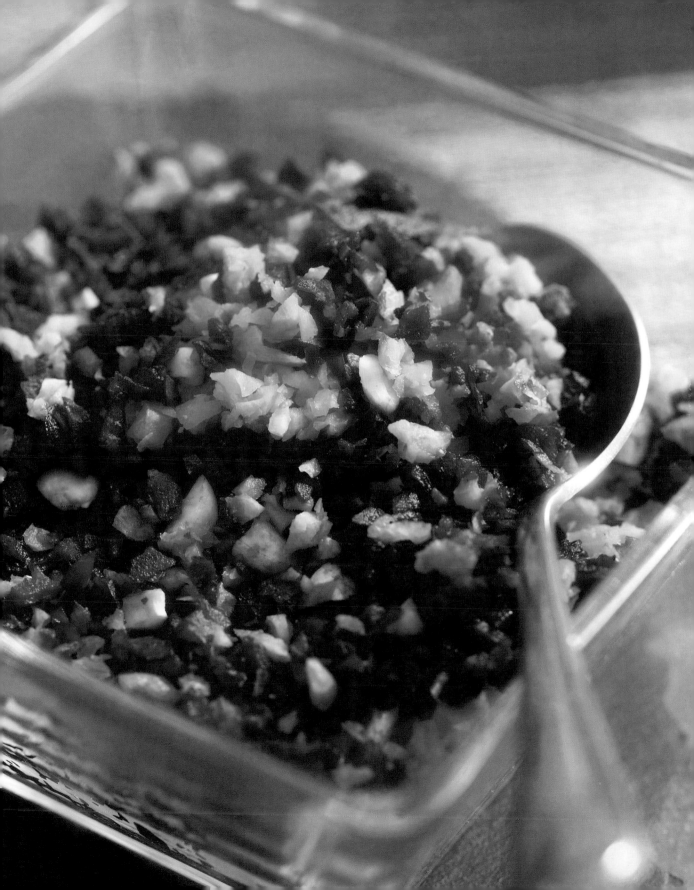

SESAME SEEDS

Lignan-Rich Super Seed

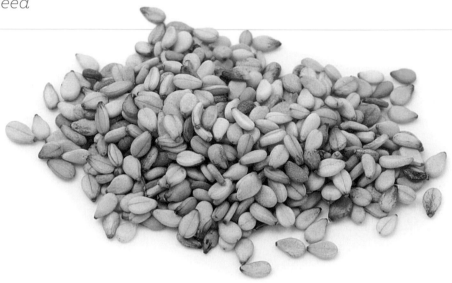

Sesame seeds are the tiny seeds found within the small pods·of an annual plant (*Sesamum indicum*) thought to be native to Africa. They have enjoyed a long history of use as food and medicine—one that spans thousands of years—and today they are cultivated around the world, including in the United States. They are packed with important nutrients and disease-fighting phytochemicals that may help promote a healthy heart and fight cancer. Adding a sprinkle of sesame seeds, a spoonful of sesame oil, or a dollop of tahini (sesame seed paste) to your diet will not only add a little flavor to your plate, but a powerful nutrient punch.

Sowing the Seeds of Good Health

Sesame seeds are an excellent source of nutrients, including heart-healthy fats, minerals, fiber, and protein. They are a good source of copper, magnesium, iron, and zinc. Although they contain substantial amounts of calcium—more than 1,400 milligrams per cup—researchers aren't sure how much of that calcium we can actually take in because of the seed's high levels of calcium-binding oxalates (compounds that prevent absorption).

Sesame seeds are also rich in fats, more than 80 percent of which are in the form of heart-healthy mono- and polyunsaturated fatty acids. And a mere tablespoon (8 g) of the seeds contains just over a gram of fiber, which may not seem like a lot but adds up to more than 11 grams per cup (144 g). A tablespoon (8 g) of sesame seeds also contain about 1.5 grams of protein—or 25 grams per cup (144 g)—more than the amount found in a chicken breast.

Good-for-Your-Heart, Cancer-Combating Super Seed

Sesame seeds are one of the two best sources of lignans (the other being flax), a group of disease-fighting phytochemicals. Two major lignans in sesame seeds, sesamin and sesamolin, have strong anti-oxidant and anti-inflammatory properties. Researchers have found that sesamin, in particular, may help reduce cholesterol levels in the blood and liver, lower triglycerides, and improve blood pressure, all of which may help reduce the risk of athero-sclerosis, stroke, and heart disease.

In a study published in 2012 in the *International Journal of Food Sciences and Nutrition*, researchers looked at the effects of sesame seed consumption on risk factors related to heart disease in thirty-eight patients with elevated lipids. After sixty days, they found that those who consumed 40 grams (about 1½ ounces) of white sesame seeds daily had significant reductions in total and LDL ("bad") cholesterol levels. Consumption of these tiny powerhouses also helped enhance antioxidant activity and reduce the oxidation of lipids (which can cause artery-clogging plaques to form).

The lignans in sesame seeds may also help prevent cancer cells from growing and spreading. In a study published in 2010, researchers at the University of Texas tested the effects of a sesame seed–derived extract of sesamin on various lines of cancer cells. They found that sesamin inhibited tumor formation of colon, prostate, breast, lung, and pancreatic cancer cells. It also re-duced the growth and proliferation of leukemia and multiple myeloma cells, causing from 9 to 69 percent and 10 to 47 percent, respectively, to self-destruct.

PUTTING IT INTO PRACTICE

Hulled or unhulled sesame seeds, tahini, and sesame oil are simple to add to your diet. Sesame seeds can be toasted (which increases their nutty flavor) and tossed into salads or baked goods. You can also purchase or make your own gomasio, a seasoning that is created by toasting sesame seeds and then grinding them with salt. Sprinkle gomasio on nearly any dish—soups, salads, and steamed vegetables, for example—in place of regular salt. Tahini, a seed butter that is commonly made from roasted and ground sesame seeds, can be used to make hummus or sauces. And sesame oil is a good oil for both health and cooking. Not only does it appear to have a beneficial effect on blood fats and blood pressure (just like the seed itself), but this antioxidant-rich oil is highly stable and has a medium smoke point, which makes it ideal for light sautéing or stir-frying.

GINGER-SESAME TOFU CABBAGE WRAPS

Sprinkling sesame seeds on this sweet and gingery dish adds a little calcium and cancer-fighting lignans to the already calcium- and protein-rich tofu. I like wrapping the soft bites of tofu in cabbage, but you can also serve over brown rice.

14 ounces (395 g) extra-firm tofu
¼ cup (60 ml) tamari
¼ cup (60 ml) mirin
3 tablespoons (45 ml) freshly squeezed lime juice
2 tablespoons (40 g) agave syrup
2 cloves garlic, crushed
1 tablespoon (8 g) grated fresh ginger
2 tablespoons (16 g) toasted sesame seeds
10 small to medium-size cabbage leaves

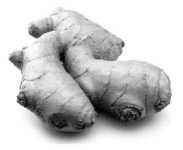

Yield: 3 to 4 servings

Preheat the oven to 350°F (180°C, or gas mark 4).

Drain the tofu, pat dry, and cube. Place the tofu cubes in a single layer in a 9 × 13-inch (23 × 33 cm) baking dish. In a small bowl, whisk together the tamari, mirin, lime juice, agave syrup, garlic, and ginger. Pour the marinade over the tofu and bake for 45 to 50 minutes, stirring occasionally.

Meanwhile, in a small, dry skillet, heat the sesame seeds over medium heat until golden, 3 to 5 minutes. Set aside.

When the tofu is done cooking, remove from the oven and let stand for 5 to 10 minutes.

Place ¼ cup (55 g) of tofu on each cabbage leaf, sprinkle with sesame seeds, and fold the leaf with the seam down. Serve warm or cold. Use any additional sauce in the pan for dipping.

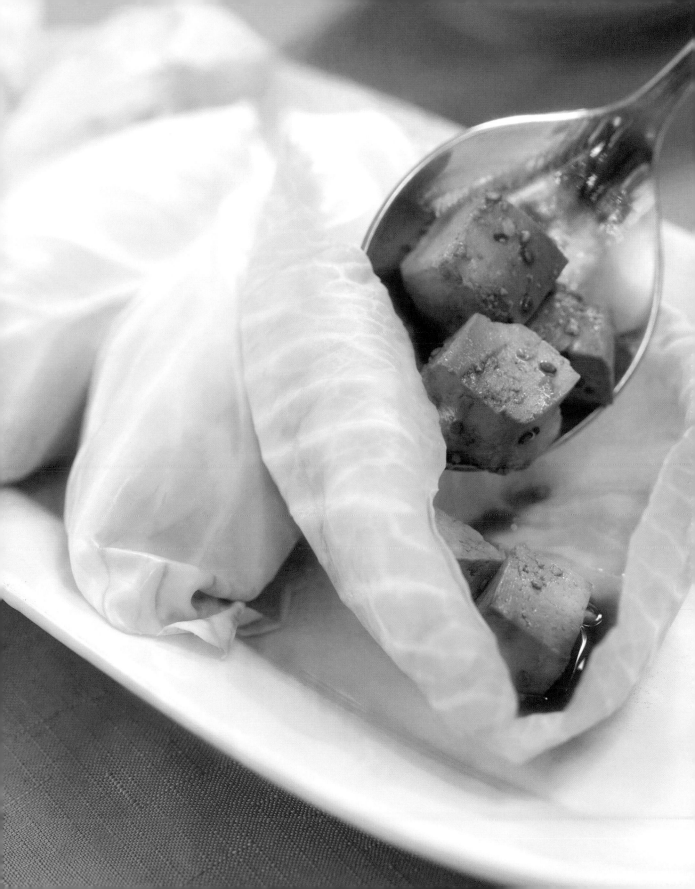

WALNUTS

King of Nuts

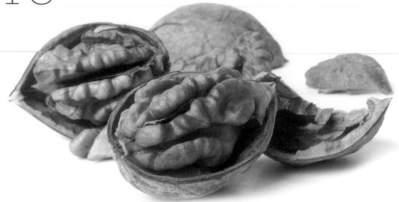

Contrary to popular belief, walnuts won't make you gain weight—and may even help you lose weight. In a 2010 review, researchers noted an inverse relationship between nut consumption and weight—meaning that higher intakes of nuts (two or more servings a week) were associated with lower body weights and body mass indexes. In addition, studies have consistently found that—despite an increase in caloric intake—walnut-enriched diets do not cause weight gain. Although nuts are thought to increase thermogenesis (the amount of calories you burn digesting the food you eat), researchers speculate that the satiety-promoting effect of the fat, protein, and fiber in walnuts helps reduce appetites and benefit weight.

Walnuts top the charts when it comes to their high levels of antioxidants and omega-3 fatty acids—in fact, no other nut comes close. These super nuts may help lower your risk of heart disease, diabetes, and cancer; and their high levels of omega-3 fatty acids will invigorate your brain (and possibly your mood). And if you think these calorie- and fat-dense nuts might pack on the pounds, think again: walnuts may actually help you stay slim. Indeed, walnuts are kings in the world of nuts and seeds—and an incredibly accessible and simple superfood to add to your diet.

An Army of Antioxidants

One ounce (28 g) of walnuts contains about 4 grams of protein, about 2 grams of fiber, and meets about 10 percent of your daily needs for bone-building magnesium and phosphorous. Walnuts are also rich in other minerals like manganese, copper, phosphorous, and magnesium. They contain impressively high levels of antioxidants including vitamin E, selenium, and polyphenols like ellagic acid (which promotes heart health and fights cancer) and melatonin

(which helps regulate sleep and wake cycles). In a study published in the *American Journal of Clinical Nutrition* in 2006, researchers examined the antioxidant content of more than one thousand foods, and they found that walnuts ranked second among all foods (only behind blackberries). And in a study published in 2012, researchers at the University of Scranton found that walnuts not only had the highest levels of polyphenols of all nuts tested (including nine different roasted and raw nuts and two types of peanut butter), but the best antioxidant activity, too (meaning they were exceptional at scavenging cell-damaging free radicals).

Walnuts Are Good for Your Heart and Blood Vessels

Walnuts contain the highest levels of omega-3 fatty acids of any nut. One ounce (28 g) of walnuts (about ¼ cup of shelled halves or pieces) contains 18 grams of fat, but more than 70 percent of that fat is in the form of polyunsaturated fatty acids, including the omega-3 alpha-linolenic acid. They also contain arginine, an essential amino acid that helps protect the heart and blood vessels. In the body, arginine is converted to nitric oxide, which helps the blood vessels relax and prevents artery-clogging platelets from accumulating.

Researchers have found that walnuts may help lower cholesterol and triglyceride levels and reduce the formation of artery-clogging plaque that can lead to heart attack and stroke. In a study published in the *American Journal of Clinical Nutrition* in 2009, researchers at Loma Linda University found that subjects who consumed a walnut-enriched diet about 1½ ounces [42.5 grams] of walnuts) over a four-week period significantly reduced their total and LDL ("bad") cholesterol levels compared to those following a fish diet about ¼ pound [113 grams], of salmon twice weekly) and a control diet (no fish or walnuts). And here's more good news for walnut-lovers: Replacing red meat with walnuts may slash your risk of type 2 diabetes. After following more than 200,000 adults from three different studies, researchers from the Harvard School of Public Health found that substituting a serving of nuts—like walnuts—each day in place of red meat can lower the risk of developing type 2 diabetes by 16 to 35 percent.

PUTTING IT INTO PRACTICE

Two types of walnuts are commonly available today: English walnuts (*Juglans regia*) and black walnuts (*Juglans nigra*). Although they are cultivated around the world, more than half of all walnuts are grown in California, where they are typically harvested from late August through November. You can buy walnuts shelled or unshelled and store them at home in a tightly lidded container at room temperature (for immediate use), or in the refrigerator (for up to 1 month) or freezer (for long-term storage).

Raw or roasted walnuts can be enjoyed alone as a snack or tossed into warm bowls of oats, quinoa, amaranth, or other cereals. They can be added to baked goods like muffins or breads, as well as salads, granolas, and trail mixes. I often use walnuts in homemade pesto sauces in place of more costly pine nuts and as a nut base for homemade raw food bars and treats.

RUSTIC APPLE CRISP

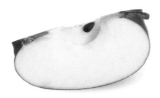

As soon as the first chilly days of fall arrive, I start making a weekly batch of this rustic apple crisp. And it's not hard to do given the bounty of ready-to-pick apples at our local orchards. Feel free to sprinkle extra walnuts in the topping for added antioxidants, omega-3 fatty acids, and crunch!

For the Topping:

1	cup (80 g) rolled oats*
½	cup (56 g) almond meal
⅓	cup (75 g) packed brown sugar
½	cup (113 g) coconut oil, room temperature (should be solid, not liquid)
½	cup (60 g) chopped walnuts

For the Filling:

2	teaspoons ground cinnamon
¼	teaspoon ground nutmeg
3	tablespoons (21 g) almond meal
8 to 10	medium-size apples, cored, peeled, and sliced thinly
2	tablespoons (40 g) pure maple syrup
1	teaspoon pure vanilla extract

Yield: 6 to 8 servings

* If you're concerned about eating gluten-free, refer to page 18 for more information on rolled oats.

Preheat the oven to 350°F (180°C, or gas mark 4). Spray a 9 × 13-inch (23 × 33 cm) baking dish with cooking spray or grease lightly with coconut oil.

To make the topping: Mix the oats, almond meal, and brown sugar together in medium-size bowl. Add the coconut oil and blend with your fingers until moist clumps form. Mix in the walnuts. Store the topping in the refrigerator while you prepare the filling.

To make the filling: Combine the cinnamon, nutmeg, and almond meal in small mixing bowl and place the sliced apples in a large mixing bowl. Whisk together the maple syrup and vanilla and drizzle over the apples, tossing to combine. Add the spice mixture to the apples and toss until the apples are evenly coated.

Place the filling in the prepared baking dish and sprinkle with the topping. Bake until the apples are tender and the top is golden brown, about 1 hour.

Allow the crisp to cool for about 10 minutes before serving. Serve warm.

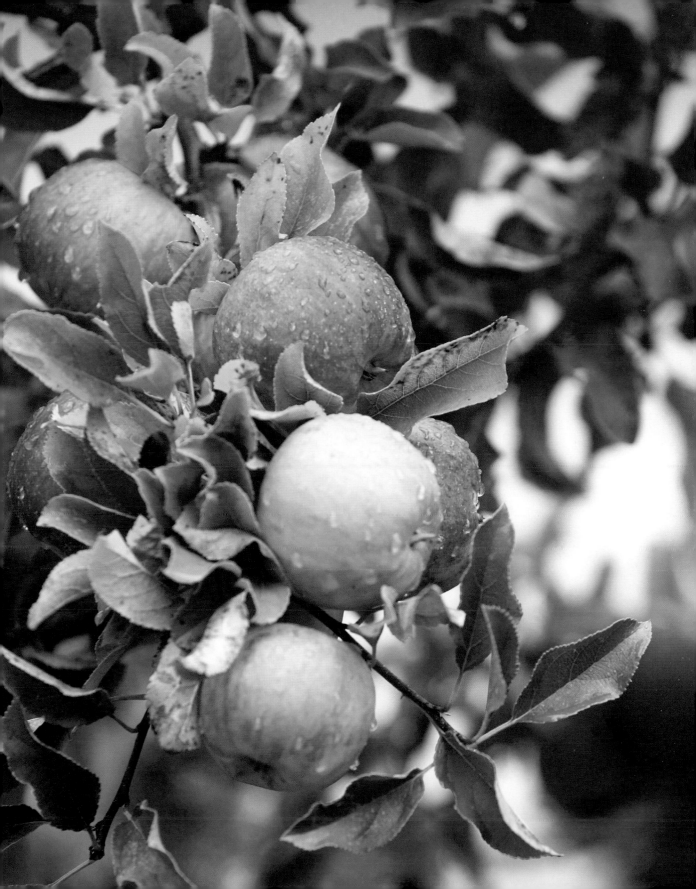

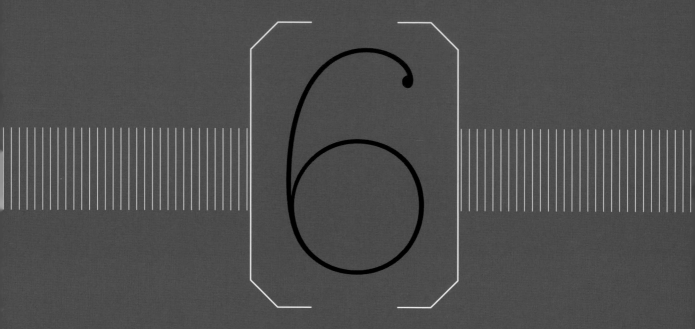

SUPER HERBS AND SPICES

Cayenne, Cinnamon, Garlic, Ginger,
Oregano, Turmeric

These powerful herbs and spices do more than just add flavor to your everyday meals. They have potent antioxidant and anti-inflammatory properties that help fight cell-damaging free radicals and inflammation. And some of the herbs and spices in this diverse group may even help you control your blood sugars, ease pain and inflammation, speed up your metabolism, and reduce your risk of chronic conditions like heart disease, diabetes, and cancer. Use these super herbs and spices liberally for flavor and health.

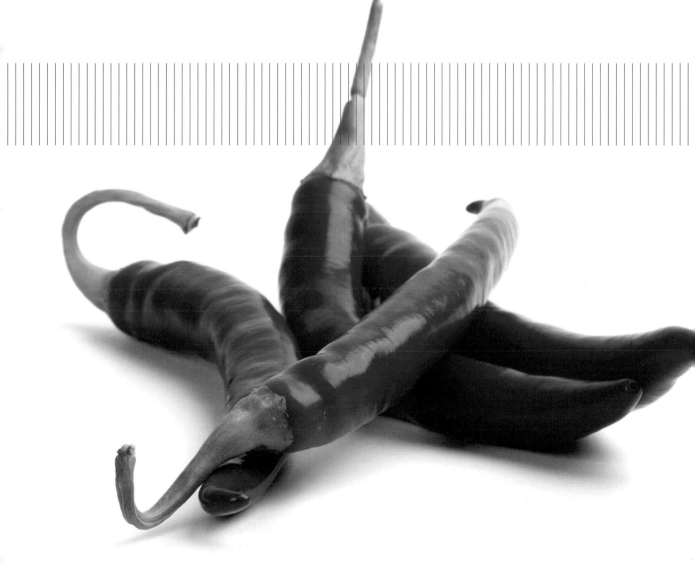

CAYENNE

Pain-Fighting Pepper

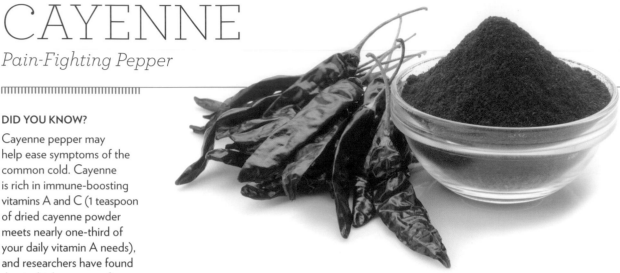

Although it has been used for thousands of years as food and medicine, cayenne pepper became quite popular a few years ago with the resurgence of the Master Cleanse diet and its copycats. After a few celebrities raved about the benefits of the cleanse—which involved drinking a homemade "lemonade" consisting of water, lemon juice, maple syrup, and cayenne pepper—droves of family members, friends, and clients began trying it in the hopes of cleansing, detoxifying, boosting metabolism, burning fat, and ultimately losing weight. I can't say for sure whether this popular cleanse delivered the results they were looking for (and I'm not so sure anyone lasted more than a day or two on it), but after doing a little research of my own, there was one thing I knew for sure: cayenne itself is one hot and spicy superfood with a host of health benefits.

Pain- and Disease-Fighting Super Spice

Cayenne peppers are the fruit of bushes (of the *Capsicum* genus) native to Central and South America, though they are currently cultivated in tropical regions around the world. Known as red peppers, hot peppers, or chile peppers, cayenne is a powerhouse of nutrients, and like most herbs and spices, it has strong antioxidant activity. Cayenne is a rich source of vitamins A and C, along with cancer-fighting carotenoids like carotenes and lutein, the latter of which promotes eye health. But cayenne is probably best known for its high content of capsaicin, a compound that gives it its intense heat and is responsible for many of its health-promoting properties. The hotter the pepper, the more capsaicin it contains—and cayenne tops the list when it comes to hot peppers (followed by jalapeños).

Capsaicin is a potent phytochemical with antioxidant, anti-inflammatory, and anticancer properties. Researchers have found that it not only helps reduce inflammation, but also serves as a natural form of pain relief for conditions like back pain, osteoarthritis, rheumatoid arthritis, nerve pain (from conditions like shingles and diabetic neuropathy), and headaches. In a study published in 2010, researchers found that patients with chronic soft tissue pain experienced a nearly 50 percent reduction in pain after using a capsaicin-based topical cream compared to those in the placebo group. When used topically, it may even help treat certain skin conditions like psoriasis (though sensitive individuals may experience side effects like burning).

And, of course, cayenne pepper is a disease-fighting super spice that reduces inflammation when taken internally. Studies have shown that its capsaicin may help reduce blood cholesterol and triglyceride levels, prevent blood clots associated with stroke and heart attack, and stop the growth and proliferation of certain cancer cells, including those of the liver, breast, prostate, brain, and skin. Researchers have also found that it may help lower blood glucose and insulin levels and improve insulin sensitivity.

DID YOU KNOW?

Spicy cayenne pepper may help you lose weight. A few studies suggest that the active compounds in cayenne peppers—including both the spicy capsaicin and nonpungent capsiate—may help you boost your metabolism, burn more calories and fat, and even suppress the accumulation of body fat, particularly in your waistline. Cayenne also appears to act as a natural appetite suppressant that may help you eat—and ultimately weigh—less.

PUTTING IT INTO PRACTICE

Cayenne peppers are most readily available as a dried powder, which can easily be added to soups and chili as well as beverages like tea, lemon water, and homemade smoothies (it is a great complement to citrus-based juices and smoothies like those that include orange or grapefruit). Adding a sprinkle of cayenne pepper to a cup of warm lemon water first thing in the morning is a great way to invigorate your metabolism and awaken digestion. You can also add cayenne pepper to hot cocoa: simply sprinkle in a pinch (about $\frac{1}{8}$ teaspoon per 16 to 24 ounces [475 to 710 ml] of beverage) for a spicy treat and jolt of inflammation-fighting nutrients. Additionally, cayenne pepper is a great complement to other food superstars: greens. Sauté a bunch of your favorite leafy greens—from kale and chard to dandelion greens and spinach—with a few sprinkles of cayenne pepper for extra flavor and nutrition.

SPICY WATERMELON CHIA FRESCA

Sweet and hydrating watermelon juice combines with the tartness of lime and spice of cayenne pepper for a refreshing beverage with a kick. For an extra-cold drink, chill the watermelon chunks prior to juicing. You can also serve over ice.

4 to 6   cups (600 to 900 g) watermelon chunks (enough to produce about 16 to 24 ounces [475 to 700 ml] of juice), seeded

3   limes, peeled
Several generous pinches of cayenne pepper

2 to 3   teaspoons (9 to 14 g) chia seeds (1 teaspoon per 8-ounce [235 ml] glass)

Push the watermelon chunks and limes through a juicer. Divide the juice between two glasses (if sharing). Sprinkle with a few generous pinches of cayenne pepper. Stir 1 to 1½ teaspoons of chia into each glass and let stand for about 10 minutes, stirring once or twice during that time. Serve chilled.

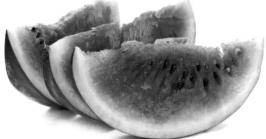

Yield: 2 servings

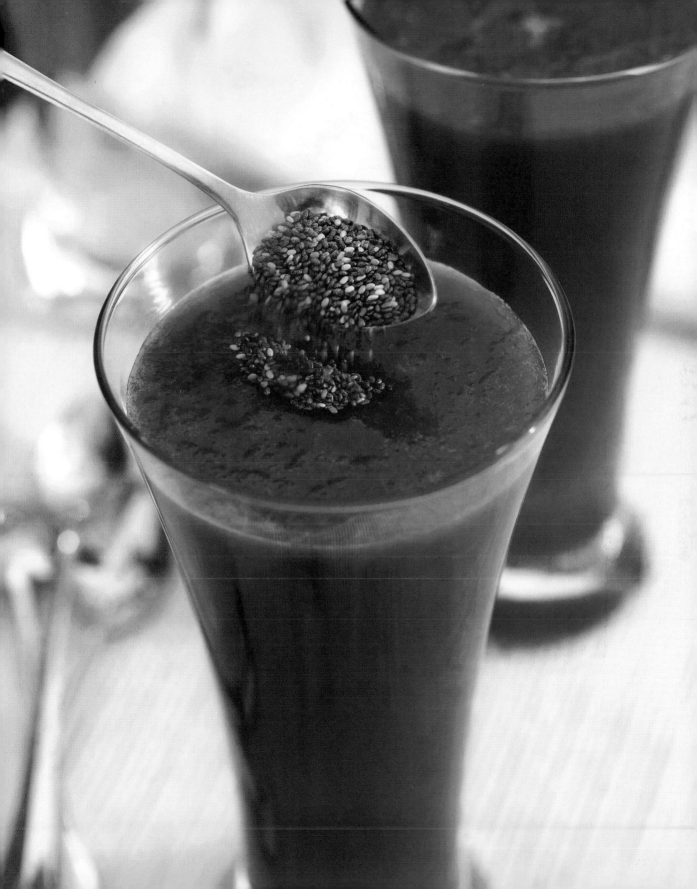

CINNAMON
Blood Sugar–Lowering Spice

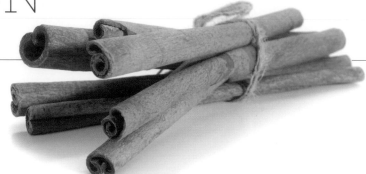

DID YOU KNOW?

When it comes to cinnamon (and a few other herbs and spices), more is not always better. You might assume that if a little bit of cinnamon could lower blood sugar and lipid levels, then a large amount might have greater benefits. Not so. Although consuming 1 to 6 grams (½ to 2½ teaspooons) of cinnamon daily appears to be safe, higher levels can actually be toxic. This is because cinnamon—in particular, cassia cinnamon—contains high levels of coumarin, a compound that acts as a blood thinner and may cause liver damage when consumed in large amounts. According to the National Center for Complementary and Alternative Medicine of the National Institutes of Health, cinnamon appears to be safe when taken by mouth in amounts of up to 6 grams (2½ teaspooons) daily for fewer than six weeks. So stick with 6 grams or less per day for health—and flavor!

Cinnamon is one of the most well-known and widely used spices in the world. It has a long history of use as food and medicine that spans thousands of years. Native to China, India, and parts of Southeast Asia, this popular spice is derived from the bark of the cinnamon tree, an evergreen of which there are hundreds of varieties. The two most common varieties of cinnamon used today are Ceylon cinnamon (*Cinnamomum zeylanicum*), also known as "true" cinnamon, and cassia cinnamon (*Cinnamomum aromaticum*), also known as Chinese cinnamon. In North America, cassia is the more popular and less expensive of the two varieties, and although researchers aren't sure whether one is nutritionally superior to the other, both appear to benefit health.

Cinnamon Improves Blood Sugar Levels

Cinnamon has been described as an anti-inflammatory, antitumor, antimicrobial, and antiviral food. It is rich in numerous active compounds including polyphenols, a large group of phytochemicals with strong antioxidant and anti-inflammatory activities that also appear to help improve insulin sensitivity. In a study published in 2000, researchers at the U.S. Department of Agriculture (USDA) examined the effects of forty-nine different herbs, spices, and medicinal extracts on glucose and insulin metabolism. They found that cinnamon had the greatest effect on insulin activity—in fact, twenty times more than all other compounds tested. With few exceptions, studies have consistently found that cinnamon helps lower blood sugars, particularly in those with type 2 diabetes.

One of the first studies examining the effects of cinnamon on the blood sugar levels of individuals with type 2 diabetes was published in 2003. In the study, sixty men and women consumed 1, 3, or 6 grams (½ to 2½ teaspoons) of cinnamon daily, divided into two doses, or were given a placebo. After forty days, researchers found that those who consumed the cinnamon experienced an 18 to 29 percent decrease in blood sugars, a 23 to 30 percent decrease in triglycerides, a 7 to 27 percent decrease in LDL ("bad") cholesterol, and a 12 to 26 percent decrease in total cholesterol. The placebo group experienced no changes. Subsequent studies have seen similar effects when it comes to cinnamon's ability to help regulate blood sugar levels.

In a study published in 2010, researchers looked at the effects of cinnamon on fifty-eight subjects with type 2 diabetes. They received either 2 grams of cinnamon (about 1 teaspoon) or a placebo daily in conjunction with their diabetes medications. Researchers found that those who took cinnamon experienced decreases in fasting blood glucose levels, waist circumference, and body mass index over a twelve-week period. Although the changes were not considered significant when compared with the placebo group, subjects treated with cinnamon did experience significant reductions in both hemoglobin A1c (a marker of long-term blood sugar control) and blood pressure. Indeed, most research supports the use of as little as 1 gram (½ teaspoon) and up to 6 grams (2½ teaspoons) of cinnamon daily to help improve blood sugar, cholesterol, LDL cholesterol, and triglyceride levels.

PUTTING IT INTO PRACTICE

Cinnamon sticks are the peeled bark from the cinnamon tree; as the bark dries, it curls up into what are called quills, and these are the cinnamon sticks that you can purchase at the market. Ground cinnamon powder is also readily available, and both the powder and sticks—not cinnamon oil—are where you will find its beneficial active compounds.

Cinnamon lends itself to warm foods and beverages, and the active components in cinnamon do not appear to be destroyed by heat. You can add a sprinkle of cinnamon or a whole cinnamon stick to warm tea or cider. I often make my own hot chocolate by simmering a cup (235 ml) or two of nondairy milk with cocoa powder and adding a whole cinnamon stick or sprinkle of ground cinnamon powder, along with a splash of pure vanilla extract and sweetener like maple syrup. Ground cinnamon also makes an excellent addition to whole-grain toast; warm cereals like buckwheat, quinoa, or oats; or applesauce.

PUMPKIN PIE QUINOA BOWL

This pumpkin bowl was inspired by the delightful warming spices used in my mom's pumpkin pie—mainly cinnamon. You can serve this sweet and creamy filling over oats, amaranth, or quinoa or enjoy the "pumpkin pie" filling on its own. It's the perfect dish to curl up with on a chilly winter morning.

½ cup (87 g) quinoa
1 cup (235 ml) water
Pinch of sea salt
2 cups (490 g) pure pumpkin puree
2 tablespoons (40 g) pure maple syrup, or more to taste
1 teaspoon pure vanilla extract
½ teaspoon lemon zest
¼ to ½ teaspoon ground cinnamon
Pinch of ground ginger
Pinch of ground nutmeg
Pinch of ground cloves

Rinse the quinoa in a strainer. Place the quinoa, water, and salt in a medium-size pot. Bring to a boil, cover, and reduce the heat until the water is absorbed, about 15 minutes.

In a separate saucepan, combine the pumpkin puree and maple syrup and heat until warmed through. Remove from the heat and add the vanilla, lemon zest, cinnamon, ginger, nutmeg, and cloves.

Fold the pumpkin puree into the quinoa and serve.

Yield: 2 to 3 servings

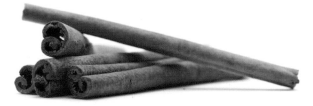

GARLIC
Nature's Wonder Drug

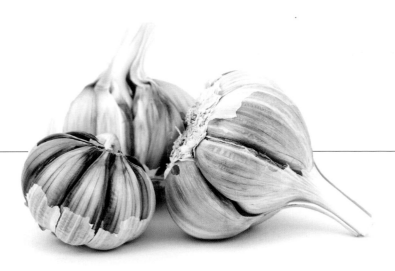

Garlic (*Allium sativum*) is a fresh herb that belongs to the Allium family, which includes onions, chives, leeks, and scallions. About three hundred different varieties of garlic are grown around the world, and most of the garlic produced in the United States is cultivated in California—though I am fortunate to have garlic farms in my own backyard here in the Finger Lakes. Garlic has long been regarded as a powerful superfood that plays a role in everything from fighting infections and boosting immunity to promoting weight loss and preventing major chronic diseases like cancer, diabetes, and heart disease.

Sulfur-Rich Super Herb

Garlic is packed with numerous antioxidants like selenium and vitamin C and heart-protecting phytochemicals like flavonoids. But it is perhaps best known for its sulfur-based compounds, which not only give garlic its unique pungent taste and odor, but are also responsible for most of its known health benefits. These compounds (including allicin, diallyl sulfide [DAS], diallyl disulfide [DADS], diallyl trisulfide [DATS],

thiacremonone, and s-allyl cysteine sulfoxide) have strong anti-inflammatory and antioxidant activities that have a protective effect on the organs. Researchers have found that these sulfur-based compounds help guard the liver, heart, intestines, lungs, brain, and kidneys from the harmful effects of heavy metals, alcohol, medications, toxins like cigarette smoke, and more. These compounds also have strong antibacterial properties that make garlic a potent infection-fighting and immune-boosting food. The allicin from garlic has been found to combat viruses and bacteria (including those of the common cold and flu), stomach viruses, yeast, and even certain strains of bacteria that are resistant to traditional antibiotic medications.

Garlic is Good for Your Heart (and Weight)

The beneficial sulfur-containing compounds in garlic may help lower total and LDL ("bad") cholesterol levels and may even help increase HDL ("good") cholesterol levels. And researchers have found that as little as one clove of garlic per day may be enough to reduce blood pressure levels, perhaps by as much as 7 to 8 percent. The flavonoids and allicin from garlic also appear to reduce blood clotting (they keep platelets from sticking together), which is an important factor in heart disease and stroke, while keeping the arteries flexible and elastic.

Garlic may also play a protective role when it comes to diabetes and obesity. A few studies have found that garlic may help lower blood sugar and insulin levels and improve insulin sensitivity. In a study published in 2011, researchers looked at the effects of raw garlic on insulin resistance and type 2 diabetes. They found that when a high-fructose diet was supplemented with raw garlic, diabetic rats experienced significant decreases in insulin resistance and blood sugar, insulin, and triglyceride levels—as well as decreases in body weight gain. And when it comes to weight, garlic just might hold the key to helping you shed excess pounds.

Several recent animal studies have found that garlic may have an anti-obesity effect in the diet, possibly due, in part, to its sulfur-containing compounds like thiacremonone, which appears to help the body burn fat and prevent the accumulation of fat in your fat cells. In a study published in 2012, researchers found that mice treated with thiacremonone over a three-week period lost weight and reduced triglyceride and blood sugar levels. In another study published in the 2011 *Journal of Nutrition*, researchers found that obese mice who consumed a 2 or 5 percent garlic-supplemented, high-fat diet for seven weeks reduced both body weight and fat stores while normalizing their levels of circulating blood and liver fats.

PUTTING IT INTO PRACTICE

Garlic is a deliciously pungent addition to the diet and readily available at supermarkets and health food stores. When purchasing, choose plump, dry heads that show no signs of browning. They can be stored in a cool, dark place, where they will last for up to about two weeks.

Crushed garlic is an excellent addition to soups, sauces, and salad dressings. I often dress my salads with a simple mixture of extra-virgin olive oil, balsamic vinegar, Dijon mustard, a clove's worth of crushed garlic, salt, and pepper. You can also roast whole heads of garlic by cutting the top of the head off to expose the cloves, drizzling with olive oil, wrapping in foil, and baking for about 45 minutes at 400°F (200°C, or gas mark 6). Roasted garlic makes a great spread or addition to soups and sauces. Garlic can also be juiced; simply wrap a clove of garlic in a leafy, green vegetable and push through the juicer.

Of course, the beneficial allicin compound is activated when garlic is broken down, so be sure to crush, chop, or mince garlic cloves and allow them to stand at room temperature for a few minutes before using. Excessive heat can destroy the beneficial sulfur compounds, so you may wish to use raw garlic in your recipes (if it does not irritate your stomach) or lightly cook it (for example, sautéing over low heat or adding to your soups and sauces toward the end of cooking time). Dried and powdered garlic is another convenient option, through drying may result in some nutrient losses.

RAW ZUCCHINI PASTA WITH PESTO SAUCE

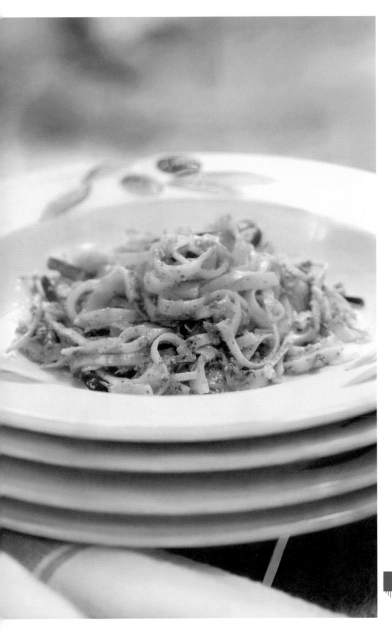

This no-cook recipe combines fresh, zucchini-based pasta with a garlicky pesto sauce. If you don't have a spiralizer to transform the zucchini into long, wavy noodles, simply use a vegetable peeler to create flat noodles for this dish.

2	medium-size zucchini, unpeeled
2	cups (48 g) tightly packed fresh basil, or 1 cup (24 g) fresh basil plus 1 cup (30 g) fresh spinach
1	cup (135 g) raw pine nuts
½	cup (120 ml) extra-virgin olive oil
2	cloves garlic, crushed
2	tablespoons (12 g) nutritional yeast
¼ to ½	teaspoon sea salt

Trim the ends of the zucchini. Peel into thin strips using a vegetable peeler for flat noodles or run through a spiralizer for long, thin, curly noodles. Place the noodles in a large mixing bowl.

For the pesto sauce, combine the basil, pine nuts, olive oil, garlic, nutritional yeast, and salt in a food processor and process until a smooth and creamy sauce forms. Pour the sauce over the noodles, toss to coat, and serve.

Yield: 3 to 4 servings

GINGER

Inflammation-Fighting Super Spice

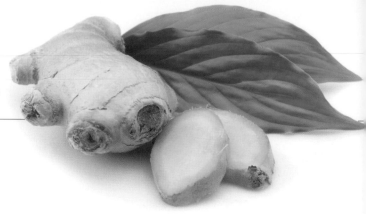

DID YOU KNOW?

Ginger may help relieve nausea and vomiting associated with pregnancy, motion sickness, surgery, and chemotherapy. Although dosages in clinical trials have varied, on average, it appears that consuming anywhere from 0.5 to 3.5 grams (¼ to 2 teaspoons) of ground ginger or 0.5 to 1.0 grams (¼ to ½ teaspoon) of fresh ginger may help in the short-term relief of nausea. For pregnant women, some initial studies have found that 1 gram (about ½ teaspoon) of ground ginger per day from anywhere from four days to three weeks may be effective. Of course, if you are pregnant, consult with your health-care provider.

When I was pregnant several years back, my acupuncturist recommended making fresh ginger tea to treat the horrible nausea and vomiting I was experiencing during my first trimester. I was skeptical at first (how could grating a little fresh ginger into hot water relieve my nausea?), but quite simply, it worked. This rhizome (underground stem), part of a perennial plant (*Zingiber officinale*) native to Asia, has been used for culinary and medicinal purposes for thousands of years. Its potent antioxidant and anti-inflammatory properties may, indeed, help calm an upset stomach and ease pain and inflammation. Researchers are also finding that ginger may improve risk factors associated with heart disease, destroy cancer cells, and even improve blood sugars. If you have an affinity for ginger as I do now (and from my experience, I have found that clients either love it or hate it), you will be happy to know that this herb is truly a superfood for super health.

Cancer Cell-Destroying Terpenes

Ginger contains numerous phytonutrients, including a group of active phenols called gingerols, which contribute not only to its pungent taste but also to its antioxidant and anti-inflammatory properties, and terpenes (like monoterpenoids and sesquiterpenoids), which are thought to have cancer-fighting potential. The many active compounds in ginger are thought to contribute to its ability to help reduce inflammation, prevent the growth and spreading of certain cancer cells, and lower high blood pressure, cholesterol, and blood sugar levels.

In a study published in 2012, researchers found that polyphenols extracted from ginger inhibited the proliferation of non-small-cell lung cancer cells, a largely incurable cancer that is challenging to treat. After ninety-six hours, researchers found that the ginger extract caused the population of cancer cells to decrease to 26 percent of its original numbers and induced apoptosis (self-destruction) by 39 percent. In another study published in 2012, researchers in China found that an extract of zerumbone, a sesquiterpene isolated from ginger, caused the self-destruction of pancreatic cancer cells. Although it is difficult to say whether the activity of extracts used in cell studies would have similar effects in the body, it is clear that ginger contains some potent cancer-fighting compounds.

A Natural Blood Thinner

Ginger appears to have blood-thinning effects similar to that of aspirin and may help prevent the accumulation of platelets that can lead to clogged arteries and increased risk of heart attack and stroke. Studies have also found that extracts of ginger may help reduce blood pressure, in part, by relaxing the blood vessels and acting as a calcium channel blocker, much like blood pressure medications that prevent calcium from entering the cells of the heart and blood vessels.

Animal studies have also found that ginger may help reduce blood cholesterol and triglyceride levels. In a study published in the *British Journal of Nutrition*, researchers found that diabetic rats whose diets were enriched with raw ginger over a seven-week period experienced significant reductions in blood glucose, cholesterol, and triglyceride levels compared with the control group that received no ginger.

Pain Relief—Without the Side Effects

Just as ginger appears to have the blood-thinning effects of aspirin, it also seems to have the same anti-inflammatory and pain-relieving properties of nonsteroidal anti-inflammatory drugs (NSAIDs) like ibuprofen—and without the negative side effects associated with NSAID use, including increased risk of stomach bleeding and ulcers. Active gingerols, shogaols, paradols, and zingerone appear to block pathways in the body that lead to inflammation and reduce the production of inflammatory compounds. And according to researchers, these actions may benefit those with osteoarthritis, rheumatoid arthritis, and musculo-skeletal pain. A few studies have found that consuming ginger in dosages of 30 to 500 milligrams daily over four to thirty-six weeks may reduce hip and knee pain in those with osteoarthritis.

In a study published in 2010, researchers at Georgia College and State University tested the effects of ginger on exercise-induced muscle pain and soreness. They found that subjects who consumed 2 grams (about 1 teaspoon) of raw or heated ginger for seven days before and three days after high-intensity eccentric weightlifting (strength exercises that emphasize the lowering phase of a movement in which the muscles lengthen—such as lowering the dumbbell during a bicep curl) had about 25 percent less muscle pain and soreness than the placebo group twenty-four hours after exercise. And according to the researchers, the amount of pain relief that subjects experienced demonstrate that ginger is at least as, if not more, effective in treating muscle soreness than traditional NSAIDs.

PUTTING IT INTO PRACTICE

If you want to add ginger to your diet, I recommend purchasing both fresh and ground ginger. Fresh ginger should be smooth, firm, and free of any mold, soft spots, or wrinkled skin. You can store unpeeled ginger in the refrigerator, where it will last for several weeks, or in the freezer for long-term storage. The skin is easily peeled off using the tip of a spoon and can be sliced, chopped, or grated into homemade ginger teas, soups, stir-fries, and vegetable dishes (one of my favorites is sweet potatoes and greens with ginger). You can also peel and juice whole ginger; it is a great accompaniment to green juices and carrot, apple, or beet blends. Ground ginger can be added to baked goods or sprinkled into warm cereals. Just remember that ground ginger has a much more pungent taste than fresh, so use sparingly.

GINGERY RED JUICE

Red juices are bright and colorful and usually much sweeter than green juices because of the addition of sweet root vegetables like beets and carrots. Ginger juice is the perfect accompaniment to these sweet vegetables, and if you enjoy the taste of fresh ginger as I do, add an extra piece or two to your juice for a big boost of flavor and inflammation-fighting compounds.

4 to 6 medium-size carrots, peeled
1 medium-size beet, peeled
¼ head cabbage
1 apple

1 lemon, peeled
1 thumb-size piece of ginger, peeled

Push all the ingredients through a juicer and serve.

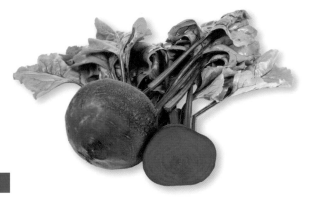

Yield: 2 servings

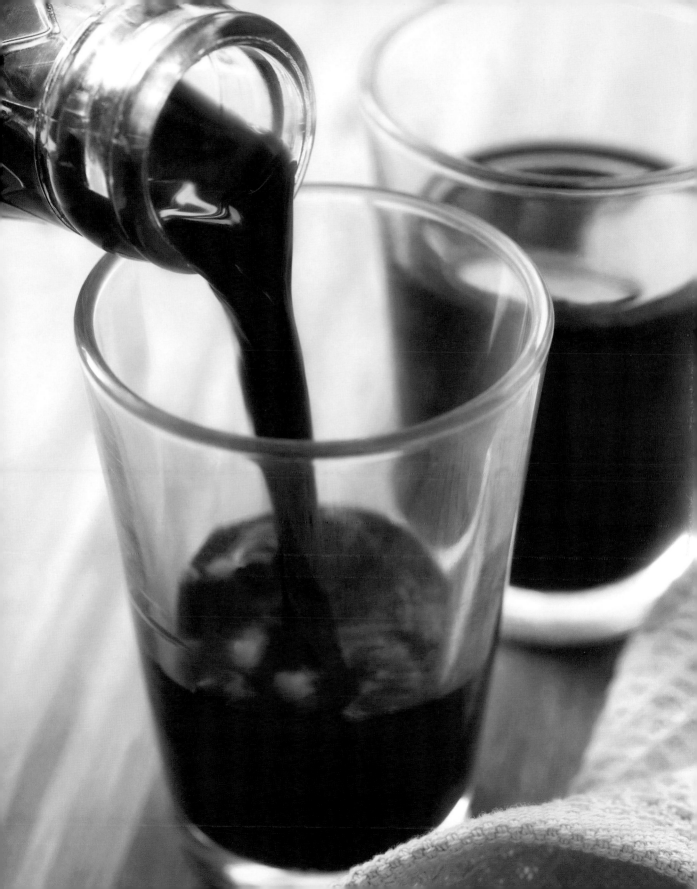

OREGANO

Antioxidant-Rich Super Herb

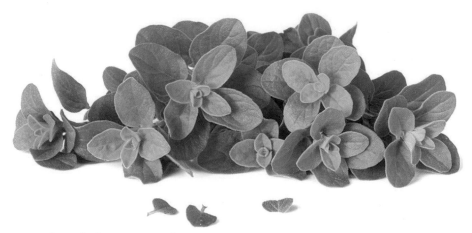

Back in the late 1990s, when I was working and living in Washington, D.C., my mother insisted I have a garden—despite the fact that I was living in a fifth-floor studio apartment with a tiny balcony. So every May for four years, she would arrive at my building with potting soil and herbs in hand and set about planting a garden along the sunny edge of my balcony. Indeed, no space was too small to grow food, and thus, my annual herb garden was born.

Among the basil, rosemary, mint, and parsley was one of my favorite herbs—and probably the most underutilized (after all, I didn't start making my own sauce until my thirties)—oregano. Used for thousands of years as food and medicine, oregano (*Origanum vulgare*) is native to Europe but now cultivated around the world.

This super herb does more than just add flavor to food. Oregano is packed with potent compounds that may help reduce oxidative stress and fight inflammation in the body.

Eases Inflammation Associated with Arthritis, Allergies, and Asthma

Oregano is rich in numerous vitamins, minerals, and phytochemicals. A teaspoon of dried oregano leaves contains small amounts of dietary fiber, vitamins A and K, and minerals like calcium and potassium. But it is oregano's high levels of antioxidants that make it a superfood of interest.

Indeed, oregano has one of the highest levels of antioxidants of all herbs and spices. In a 2005 study published in the *Journal of Agricultural and Food Chemistry*, researchers examined the antioxidant activity of twenty-six common spices—and oregano came out on top. Researchers have found that its antioxidant compounds—including thymol, carvacrol, and rosmarinic acid— are excellent at scavenging cell-damaging free radicals and protecting cells from DNA damage. These compounds also appear to have strong antimicrobial activities, acting against certain strains of viruses and bacteria, including those implicated in ear infections and gum disease.

And the active compounds in oregano may also help fight inflammation, in part, by blocking the actions of pro-inflammatory enzymes in the body. In animal studies, researchers have found that extracts of rosmarinic acid, the most abundant phenol in oregano (and also found in rosemary and mint), reduced inflammation associated with arthritis, allergies, and asthma.

Anticancer Herb Helps Improve Blood Lipids and Sugars

Researchers have found that extracts of oregano—and some of its constituents, like carvacrol—may prevent platelets from clumping together and sticking to the walls of blood vessels (preventing clots that can lead to heart attack and stroke). They may also help lower total cholesterol and triglyceride levels and improve blood sugars and insulin sensitivity. In a study published in 2004, researchers found that diabetic rats who received a daily dose of an oregano leaf extract experienced significant decreases in blood sugar levels, suggesting that this spice has antihyperglycemic activity.

The compounds in oregano, such as rosmarinic acid and carvacrol, also seem to have anticancer activity. In cell studies, researchers have found that these compounds help protect cells from DNA damage, activate detoxification pathways in the liver, and prevent the growth and spreading of certain cancer cells, such as melanoma.

PUTTING IT INTO PRACTICE

Oregano is a super fresh herb that is full of flavor. It is one of the simplest herbs to cultivate at home in a vegetable and herb garden or in pots. You can also purchase dried or fresh oregano at your local farmers' market, supermarket, or health food store.

Oregano goes well with both tomato- and garlic-based dishes. I use oregano almost exclusively in making red sauce, which I top on vegetable pizzas, pastas, or vegetables. I use fresh oregano from the garden during the summer months and dried oregano during the winter. As a general rule of thumb, substitute 1 teaspoon of fresh oregano for ½ teaspoon of dried oregano, as the dried spice has a much stronger flavor than the fresh oregano leaves.

JOSEPHINE'S RED SAUCE

This sauce recipe has been handed down for at least three generations. It is the original sauce recipe that my grandmother Josephine made—and it combines an abundance of healthful herbs and spices, including oregano, parsley, and bay leaves. Enjoy this thick and rich sauce on pasta, vegetable pizza, or tossed with strands of spaghetti squash (my favorite way to serve it).

2 to 3   tablespoons extra-virgin olive oil

1   clove garlic, crushed

1   small onion, chopped

1   can (6 ounces [170 g]) tomato paste

4   cans (28 ounces [785 g] each) crushed tomatoes

Pinch of sugar

2   teaspoons dried parsley, or 1 tablespoon plus 1 teaspoon (5 g total) chopped fresh parsley

2   teaspoons dried oregano, or 1 tablespoon plus 1 teaspoon (5 g total) chopped fresh oregano

2   dried bay leaves, whole

Sea salt and freshly ground pepper, to taste

Place the oil in a large pot and add the garlic and onion. Stir while cooking over medium-high heat until the onion is soft, about 3 minutes. Add the tomato paste and stir for 1 minute. Add the crushed tomatoes, sugar, parsley, oregano, bay leaves, and salt and pepper, to taste. Continue to heat until the sauce begins to bubble, lower the heat, and simmer covered, for about 1 hour, stirring occasionally. Remove bay leaves before serving.

Yield: 12 cups

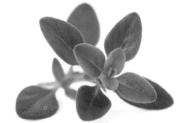

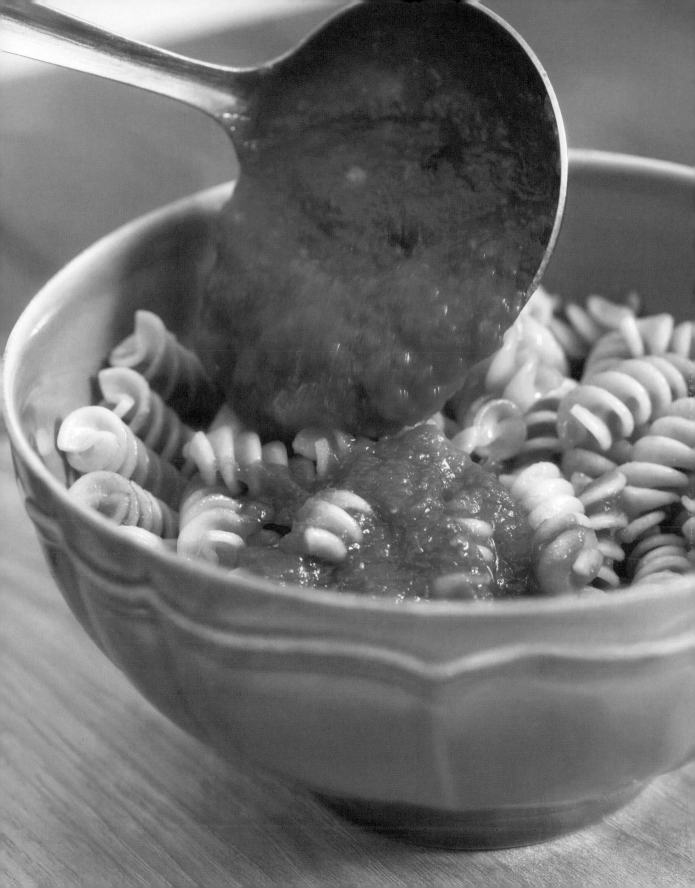

TURMERIC

Inflammation-Fighting Super Spice

DID YOU KNOW?

Turmeric may help relieve joint pain. In a study published in 2009 in the *Journal of Alternative and Complementary Medicine*, researchers compared the effects of 800 milligrams per day of ibuprofen to 2 grams per day of curcumin extracts in more than one hundred patients with osteoarthritis. After six weeks, they found that both groups experienced significant improvements in pain and joint function—with the curcumin extract being just as effective as ibuprofen.

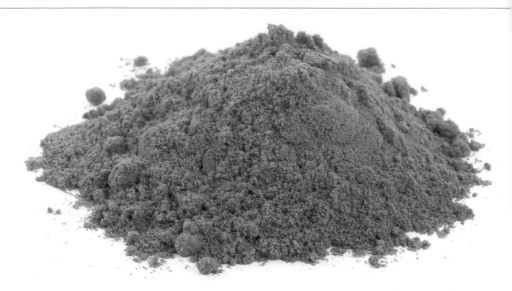

Turmeric is a spice produced from the rhizome (underground stem) of a perennial plant (*Curcuma longa*) native to Asia. It has a long history of use as both a culinary and medicinal spice and contains compounds that not only lend a strong flavor and bright yellow color to dishes like curry, but have powerful antioxidant and anti-inflammatory properties. Turmeric has been used in both Traditional Chinese and Ayurvedic medicine to decrease inflammation, heal the digestive tract, and treat skin diseases and wounds. Today, researchers are discovering that the active compounds in turmeric— mainly curcumin—may indeed help prevent or treat conditions influenced by inflammation—from age-related brain diseases and arthritis to cancer and heart disease—making it a spice worthy of superfood status.

Curcumin-Rich Spice

Turmeric contains a polyphenol called curcumin, which is a member of the curcuminoid family of compounds. Curcumin is a potent antioxidant with impressive free radical–scavenging abilities and a powerful anti-inflammatory agent that helps block the pathways that lead to inflammation while lowering levels of inflammation-producing compounds. As a result, researchers have found that curcumin may protect organs like the brain, liver, and heart; reduce inflammation associated with arthritis; lower the risk of cancer; and reduce risk factors associated with both heart disease and diabetes.

Researchers have found that curcumin-rich turmeric may also improve blood sugars and blood lipids and prevent the development of artery-clogging plaques that can lead to atherosclerosis (hardening of the arteries). Curcumin also helps remove toxins from the body and render harmless potentially cancer-causing substances. Researchers have found that it may help prevent the growth and spreading of certain cancers, including those of the prostate, breast, colon, and skin.

Curcumin's anti-inflammatory effects can also be seen in the gut, where it appears to alleviate symptoms associated with irritable bowel disease, Crohn's disease, and ulcerative colitis. And studies suggest its antibacterial properties may help reduce levels of *Helicobacter pylori*, a common stomach bacterium associated with gastritis, ulcers, and stomach cancer. When used topically, curcumin may even help ease symptoms of psoriasis and other skin conditions.

Turmeric May Help Prevent Alzheimer's Disease (and Boost Mood)

Researchers have found that curcumin-rich turmeric crosses the blood-brain barrier, where it prevents brain-clogging proteins (beta-amyloids) from collecting and forming plaques that can lead to decreased brain function and Alzheimer's disease. In a study published in 2008, researchers looked at the effects of curcumin in twenty-seven patients with Alzheimer's. After six months, they found that individuals in the curcumin group had higher blood levels of beta-amyloids, suggesting that these brain-damaging proteins were being cleared from the brain and sent into circulation.

Curcumin may also benefit those with depression. Researchers have found that it may inhibit the activity of monoamine oxidase, an enzyme involved in removing certain "feel-good" chemicals (like norepinephrine, serotonin, and dopamine) from the brain—much in the way that antidepressant medications like MAO inhibitors would. As a result, it makes these "feel-good" chemicals available to the brain, improving the communication between brain cells and boosting mood.

PUTTING IT INTO PRACTICE

Because many of the studies involving turmeric have been conducted on its main compound, curcumin, it is challenging to say just how much turmeric you would need to consume for its health benefits. As with any spice, I recommend increasing your intake of turmeric—and the other important antioxidant compounds in curcumin—by including the spice (not the supplement) in your diet. You can buy ground turmeric and add it to soups, stews, and rice and bean casseroles; sprinkle it on eggs or tofu; or make your own curry powder. You can also sip this super spice by creating a simple turmeric tea, like the recipe that follows.

NOURISHING TURMERIC TEA

DID YOU KNOW?

Adding freshly ground black pepper to turmeric-containing foods may enhance the bioavailability of curcumin. Researchers have found that in the body, curcumin is readily broken down into metabolites that may not offer up the same level of benefits as curcumin itself. However, black pepper contains a compound called piperine that seems to increase the bioavailability of curcumin (it prevents it from being metabolized too quickly). Sprinkling a little freshly ground black pepper on your next dish may help you soak up more of turmeric's health-promoting compounds and therapeutic effects.

This is a creamy and subtly spicy tea, despite the addition of a full teaspoon of two super spices. Be sure to strain this tea before drinking, and go ahead and add a sprinkle of black pepper, as researchers have found it may enhance the bioavailability of curcumin.

2 cups (475 ml) almond milk or other nondairy milk

½ teaspoon ground turmeric

½ teaspoon ground ginger

Pinch of freshly ground black pepper, to taste

Pure maple syrup

Heat the milk in a saucepan over medium heat. When hot (but not boiling), stir in the turmeric, ginger, and black pepper. Simmer uncovered for 10 minutes, stirring occasionally. Remove from the heat and strain into a coffee cup. Stir in the maple syrup to taste and serve warm.

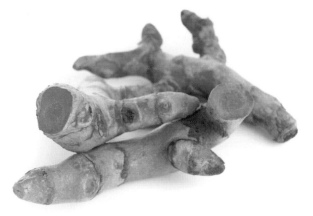

Yield: 1 to 2 servings

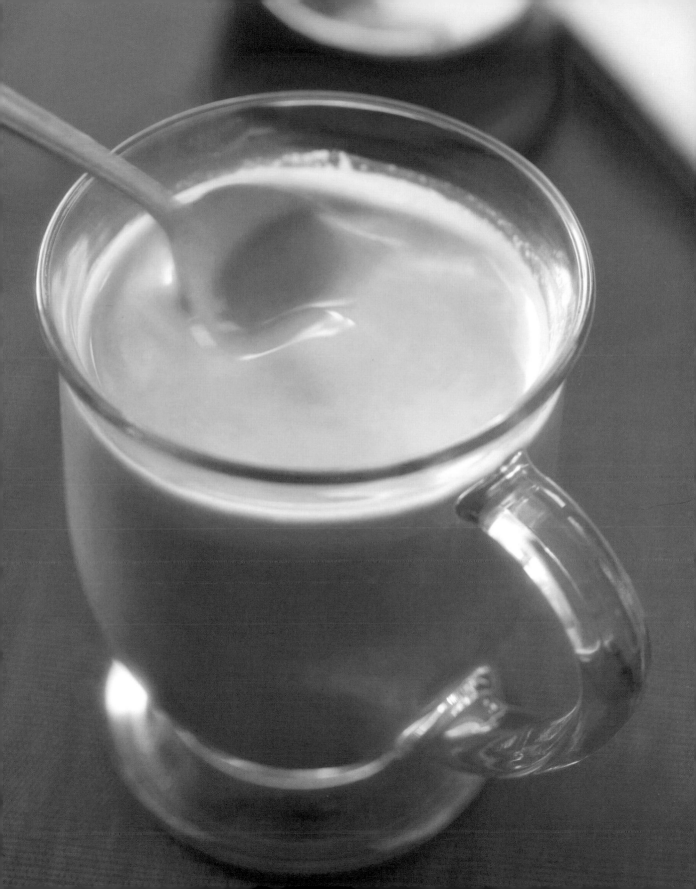

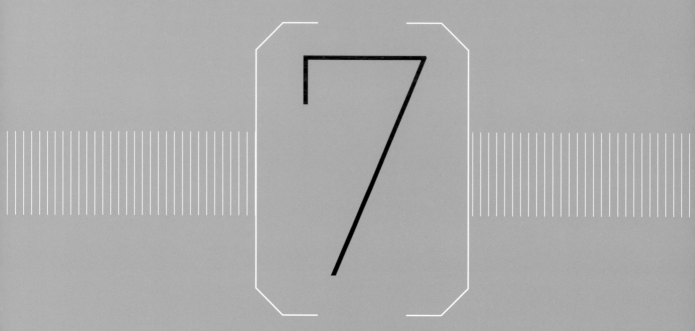

SUPER TONICS

Aloe Vera, Green Tea,
Wheatgrass Juice, Vinegar

When I think of a tonic, I think of a drink or elixir that provides nourishment and a sense of well-being. And when I looked up "tonic" in the Merriam-Webster online dictionary, it said, "One that invigorates, restores, refreshes, or stimulates." Indeed, the small group of super tonics in this chapter provides a quick and accessible way to get a boost of health-promoting compounds—after all, you simply drink them. From the healing benefits of aloe and cancer-fighting effect of green tea to the potential blood-sugar lowering ability of vinegar and energy lift from wheatgrass, you can sip your way to good health.

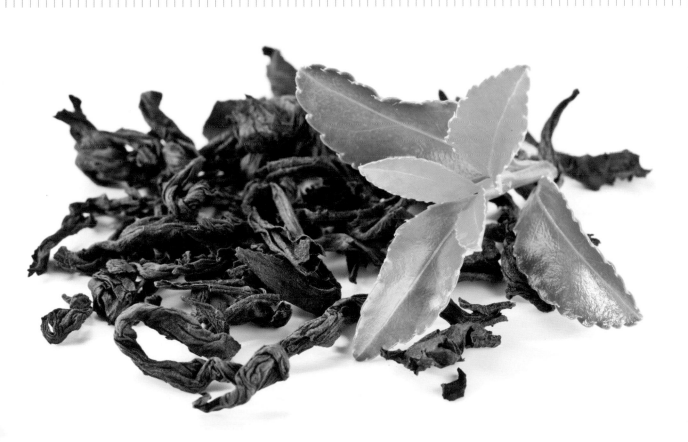

ALOE VERA
Super Healing Tonic

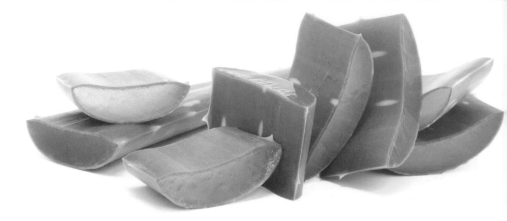

SPOTLIGHT: ALOE LATEX

Aloe latex is a yellow substance located just under the skin of the aloe leaf. It is rich in compounds like aloin, aloe-emodin, and barbaloin and has a strong laxative effect. Although aloe latex may help alleviate constipation, it can be toxic when consumed in excess or used for an extended length of time. Researchers have also found that the chemicals in aloe latex are potentially cancer-causing, can increase irritation in the intestines, and stress the liver and kidneys. And because many people develop a tolerance for aloe latex when used as a laxative, they often have to consume increasingly higher doses just to obtain the same effect. Although the U.S. Food and Drug Administration banned the inclusion of aloe in over-the-counter laxative supplements in 2002, many aloe vera products (particularly those made from the whole aloe leaf) contain aloe latex. If you choose to consume aloe gel or juice, select only those products labeled for internal consumption and avoiding those that contain aloe latex or aloin.

Aloe is a cactuslike, perennial succulent that is cultivated around the world. Researchers estimate that there are about 420 different species of plants belonging to the *Aloe* genus, of which *Aloe barbadensis*, also known as aloe vera, is the most common. Aloe vera gel, which is the clear, mucilaginous gel located in the aloe leaf, has traditionally been used as a topical ointment to heal wounds and skin conditions. It has also been taken orally to help relieve constipation, boost immunity, and treat conditions like diabetes and high blood pressure. The research on aloe is growing, and studies are finding that aloe has a vast number of nutrients and phytonutrients that play an important role in health and healing.

Internal and External Healing Properties

Aloe contains more than seventy-five vitamins, minerals, enzymes, and phytochemicals, including immune-boosting polysaccharides, inflammation-fighting salicylic acids, and aloesin, a compound thought to have potent free radical–scavenging abilities. Perhaps the most common use of aloe vera gel is in the topical treatment of wounds and skin conditions like sunburn, abrasions, dermatitis, and even psoriasis. How it heals wounds is not entirely clear, but researchers have found that aloe vera gel has noteworthy anti-bacterial and anti-fungal properties. When used topically, it may help decrease infection, reduce inflammation (and accompanying pain, itching, and burning), and even increase blood flow to the affected area to promote healing.

Just as aloe vera can help with external healing, it may also help mend the mucus lining of the intestinal tract when taken orally. Researchers have found that aloe vera gel and certain extracts of aloe may help treat oral mucositis (inflammation of the mucus membranes of the mouth, usually as a result of chemotherapy), reduce bacteria in the mouth that can contribute to tooth decay and gingivitis, and ease the symptoms of irritable bowel syndrome or ulcerative colitis.

Aloe May Help Improve Blood Sugars and Lipids

Several studies over the past decade have found that dietary aloe may help improve insulin sensitivity, reduce blood sugars and lipids, and even reduce inflammation associated with obesity. In a randomized, double-blind, placebo-controlled study published in 2012, researchers looked at the effects of aloe gel on type 2 diabetic patients with elevated blood lipids who were not responding to their current diabetes medications. Patients who took 300 milligrams of aloe gel twice daily for two months had significantly lower levels of fasting blood glucose, hemoglobin A1c (a marker of long-term blood sugar control), and total and LDL ("bad") cholesterol levels compared to the placebo group—and without any reported adverse effects.

DID YOU KNOW?

Aloe plants are simple to grow at home and provide access to an incredible healing salve: aloe vera gel. To access the gel of the fresh plant, simply cut off one of the bottom leaves close to the main stalk, trim the pointy spines along the edge, split lengthwise to reveal the clear gel, which can be scraped with the edge of a spoon, and apply topically. Although some individuals consume fresh aloe vera gel directly from the plant, I discourage it. Obtaining pure gel that is not contaminated with aloe latex is challenging.

PUTTING IT INTO PRACTICE

Bottled aloe vera gels and juices are widely available in most supermarkets and health food stores, and the best way to enjoy the benefits of mildly pungent-tasting aloe is to add an ounce (28 ml) or two of gel or juice to water, smoothies, or freshly pressed juices. What is the difference between aloe vera gel (for consumption) and aloe vera juice? The gel consists of the clear gel within the aloe leaf, whereas the juice is typically made from the whole aloe vera leaf, which is crushed and pressed to extract a juice that may then undergo filtration. If you want to add either to your diet, select products labeled for internal—not topical—use. And remember to seek out only reputable brands whose products are tested free of potentially harmful aloe latex or aloin.

ALOE WATERMELON COOLER

I usually add a splash of aloe vera juice to a tall glass of water and sip it throughout the day. However, a few summers ago, I started adding it to frozen cucumber and watermelon drinks. The mildly bitter taste of aloe combines well with sweet watermelon—creating a refreshing drink for health and healing.

1 cup (235 ml) filtered water (plus more to thin, if needed)

2 cups (300 g) watermelon, seeded and cubed

1 small cucumber, peeled and sliced

2 cups (455 g) crushed ice

2 tablespoons (28 ml) aloe vera juice (aloin-free)

Juice of 1 lime

1 tablespoon (20 g) agave syrup

3 fresh mint leaves

Pinch of sea salt

Combine all the ingredients in a high-speed blender and enjoy.

Yield: 2 servings

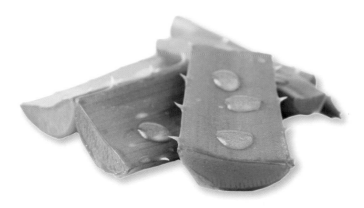

GREEN TEA
Catechin-Rich Super Tea

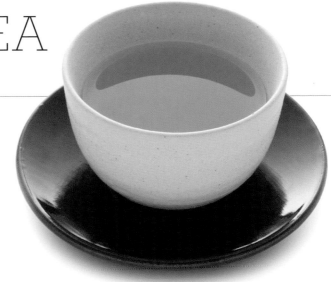

SUPERFOOD KITCHEN TIP: SQUEEZE SOME LEMON INTO YOUR TEA

The amount of beneficial polyphenols in a cup of green tea depends on the amount of tea you use, brewing time, and temperature of the water. But you can boost the bioavailability of the polyphenols in green tea—specifically, the catechins—by adding a squeeze of lemon juice to your tea. Researchers at Purdue University found that although catechins are highly unstable (it seems that less than 20 percent remain after digestion), adding citrus juice to green tea—particularly lemon juice—preserves about 80 percent of these valuable compounds. So go ahead and add a big squeeze of lemon juice to your green tea—and get ready to soak up more of its most potent antioxidants.

Tea (including black, oolong, and green) is produced from the leaves of the *Camellia sinensis* plant, a woody shrub that is native to China but produced in at least thirty countries around the world. And after water, tea is the most commonly consumed beverage worldwide. Twenty percent of all tea produced is green tea, and unlike black and oolong teas, whose leaves are fermented, the fresh leaves used to produce green tea are steamed, which helps preserve their rich content of antioxidants. In fact, green tea has one of the highest antioxidant concentrations of all teas (outside of white tea), which is the likely reason behind its ability to help fight cancer and heart disease, protect the brain and skin, and even promote fat-burning and weight loss.

Cancer-Combating Catechins

The power of green tea lies in its powerful concentration of catechins, a group of flavonoids that belong to the larger class of polyphenols. Catechins, which are also found in red wine, dark chocolate, and grapes, are associated with healthy lungs and a lower risk of heart disease and certain cancers. Green tea is particularly high in one catechin called epigallocatechin-3-gallate (EGCG), which has strong antioxidant and anti-inflammatory activities. Fifty to 75 percent of the catechins in a cup of brewed green tea consist of EGCG, and these compounds are thought to play a major role in green tea's ability to prevent and treat disease. Indeed, they may reduce the inflammation associated with Crohn's disease and ulcerative colitis, reduce oxidative stress in the brain that can lead to Alzheimer's and Parkinson's disease, and may even help fight cancer.

In cell studies, EGCG-rich extracts of green tea have been found to inhibit the growth of and destroy certain cancer cells, including those of the esophagus, breast, lung, and prostate. And in population studies, green tea consumption is, in general, associated with a reduced risk of certain cancers. One review found that increasing daily intake of green tea by 2 cups (475 ml) could decrease lung cancer risk by 18 percent, while another found that women who drank 2 or more cups of green tea each day had a 46 percent lower risk of ovarian cancer than did those who didn't. In China, studies have found that the more green tea subjects drank, the lower their risk of developing certain cancers like those of the stomach, pancreas, prostate, and esophagus.

Green Tea: Good for the Heart—and Weight

Green tea may also help improve some of the risk factors associated with heart disease and diabetes. The polyphenols in green tea appear to have blood sugar- and lipid-lowering effects, and some studies suggest that drinking 3 cups (700 ml) of green tea each day may lower the risk of heart disease. Adding green tea to your diet may also—although modestly—boost metabolism and fat burning and reduce body weight.

In a study published in 2010, researchers looked at the effects of green tea on body weight in obese subjects with metabolic syndrome. Over eight weeks, they found that subjects who consumed 4 cups (946 ml) of green tea per day had significant decreases in body weight, body mass index (a weight-to-height ratio), LDL ("bad") cholesterol levels, and certain markers of oxidative stress compared to the control group. And in a review published in 2011, researchers noted that consuming green tea catechins in the amount of 270 to 1,200 milligrams per day may help reduce body weight and fat. A cup (235 ml) of green tea contains about 200 milligrams of catechins, so this would be the equivalent of sipping more than one and up to 6 cups (1,425 ml or 1.4 L) each day.

Although drinking green tea appears to reduce body weight, researchers are often quick to point out that the results are fairly modest. In a 2010 review published in the *American Journal of Clinical Nutrition*, University of Connecticut researchers analyzed the results of more than a dozen studies on green tea and found that green tea catechins with caffeine do, indeed, reduce waist circumference, BMI, and body weight—but only an average of 2.2 pounds (1 kilogram) over a twelve-week period compared to caffeine-matched controls.

PUTTING IT INTO PRACTICE

Green tea can be purchased as whole leaf loose tea or in tea bags. I personally enjoy using whole leaf tea, but I often travel with tea bags for convenience. No matter which type of tea you prefer, store it in a tightly lidded container or tea tin in a cool, dry place.

One of the most common complaints I hear from clients regarding green tea is how bitter-tasting it is. When brewed properly, green tea is far from bitter. I recommend heating the water until just before it is ready to boil and steeping the tea leaves for a short period of time—no more than one minute. If you prefer a stronger flavor to your green tea as I do, the key is to simply use more green tea (an extra scoop of loose leaves or an extra tea bag), but keep the water temperature and brewing time the same. The longer you brew your tea, the more bitter it will become.

MATCHA GREEN TEA COOLER

I love blending frozen grapes with sparkling water or kombucha (a fermented beverage) to create a refreshing summertime drink. In this recipe, I add antioxidant-rich matcha green tea, a fine powder made from crushed green tea leaves. The combination of grapes, limes, and green tea will enhance your intake of cancer-fighting and heart-healthy polyphenols, while kombucha will flood your digestive tract with gut-friendly probiotics.

16 ounces (475 ml) kombucha
 2 cups (300 g) green grapes, frozen
    Juice of 2 limes
 2 teaspoons matcha green tea powder

Combine all the ingredients in a high-speed blender and enjoy.

Yield: 2 servings

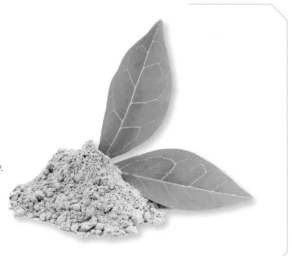

WHEATGRASS JUICE
Super Green Tonic

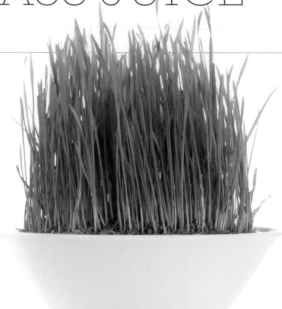

Wheatgrass is technically considered gluten free but may not be safe for those with celiac disease. Although the gluten protein is found within the seeds of the grass—not the blades of grass used to produce wheatgrass juice—there is the possibility that wheatgrass can become contaminated with seeds during production. For this reason, I recommend that individuals with celiac disease avoid consuming wheatgrass juice—and look to fresh leafy greens (juice or blended into a smoothie)—to help boost their intake of greens and beneficial nutrients.

Wheatgrass is the young, nutrient-rich grass of the wheat plant (*Triticum aestivum*) that is harvested seven to ten days after its seeds have sprouted. Although the grass itself is too fibrous to consume, fresh juice can be extracted from the leaves for its vital vitamins, minerals, antioxidants, enzymes, and phytonutrients. Wheatgrass has been a popular health food for decades, touted for its ability to do everything from treating chronic fatigue and cancer to improving digestion and blood pressure. Some advocates even claim that drinking wheatgrass juice can prevent your hair from turning gray. Although the number of health claims surrounding wheatgrass juice far outweighs the scientific evidence to support them, its decades-long history of use combined with the emergence of several new and promising scientific studies makes wheatgrass juice a super-food worth watching (and drinking).

Chlorophyll-Rich Super Grass

Wheatgrass juice contains numerous vitamins, including vitamins A, C, E, and K, and the energy-producing and stress-reducing B-complex vitamins. It is also rich in important minerals like iron, calcium, and magnesium, and contains small amounts of amino acids (the building blocks of protein). Like other green foods, wheatgrass juice is a concentrated source of chlorophyll, a pigment that gives plants their green color. Researchers have found that this important compound is able to bind with potentially cancer-causing compounds and toxins in the body, preventing their absorption. It also appears to decrease the activity of enzymes involved in activating cancer-causing chemicals.

In recent years, researchers have also identified numerous heart-healthy and cancer-fighting phytochemicals in wheatgrass juice, including flavonoids, triterpenoids, alkaloids, sterols, and tannins. And cell studies have shown that this super tonic appears to have strong antioxidant activity—both in its fresh and dried forms—as evidenced by its ability to effectively scavenge free radicals.

Lipid-Lowering, Cancer-Fighting Potential

Recent animal and cell studies have found that wheatgrass juice may help lower blood lipids and destroy certain cancer cells. In a study published in 2008, researchers from India found that healthy rats fed fresh wheatgrass juice (in doses of 5 milliliters and 10 milliliters per kilogram [2¼ pounds] of body weight) over a three-week period experienced significant and dose-dependent reductions in total cholesterol, triglyceride, LDL cholesterol, and VLDL (very-low-density lipoprotein) cholesterol levels compared to the control group.

And in 2011, researchers found similar lipid-lowering effects of wheatgrass juice when administered to rats with high cholesterol.

Researchers are also just beginning to learn about the potential anti-cancer effects of wheatgrass. In a study published in 2011, researchers found that although wheatgrass juice had no adverse effects on normal cells, it helped stop the growth and proliferation of a cancerous line of leukemia cells, causing them to self-destruct. Researchers found that wheatgrass reduced those cell numbers by 65 to 90 percent, seventy-two hours after treatment. Additionally, a study published

PUTTING IT INTO PRACTICE

Adding wheatgrass juice to your diet is incredibly simple. You can grow your own fresh wheatgrass at home (see Resources, page 215) or purchase fresh wheatgrass juice from your health food store or supermarket. You can juice the grass at home with a specialized wheatgrass juicer or masticating juicer (it will not juice well in centrifugal juicers). The juice has a mild, grassy flavor—almost reminiscent of green tea—and can be enjoyed "straight up" or mixed into other freshly pressed juices or blended smoothies.

If fresh wheatgrass juice is challenging to find or you don't want to invest in a special juicer, you can also purchase frozen wheatgrass juice—typically in the form of 1- or 2-ounce (28 to 55 g) cubes that can be thawed and consumed or dried wheatgrass powders that can be mixed into freshly-pressed juices and smoothies. I often purchase packets of dried wheatgrass and other green powders as a convenient source of greens when I am traveling.

Although some proponents claim that drinking an ounce (28 ml) of wheatgrass juice will provide the same amount of nutrients as a pound (455 g) of vegetables, I have not been able to confirm that claim. However, adding an ounce (28 ml) or two of wheatgrass juice to your weekly or daily diet—in the form of freshly extracted juice, frozen juice, or dried powder—will give you a nice boost of beneficial antioxidants and other active compounds.

Most experts recommend about ¼ to 1 teaspoon (1 to 6 grams) daily for health benefits.

in *Nutrition and Cancer* in 2007—found that wheatgrass juice supplementation (about 2 ounces [60 ml] per day) may offset some of the negative side effects of chemotherapy in patients with breast cancer.

In addition, wheatgrass juice may also ease digestion and inflammation caused by irritable bowel diseases like colitis. In a small study published in 2002, researchers found that patients with ulcerative colitis who drank about 3 ounces (90 ml) of wheatgrass juice daily for one month had decreased intestinal pain, diarrhea, and rectal bleeding compared to the control group.

APPLE SPINACH WHEATGRASS JUICE

I usually enjoy a shot or two of wheatgrass juice—straight up—a few times a week. But I also enjoy blending wheatgrass juice in other green drinks. At home, my favorite way to enjoy wheatgrass is simple: add it to fresh pressed apple juice blended with a few large handfuls of spinach. Although packed with greens, this juice is surprisingly sweet!

4 to 6	apples, juiced (enough to produce at least 12 ounces [355 ml] of juice)
2	ounces (60 ml) wheatgrass juice
2	large handfuls fresh spinach

Combine the juices and spinach in a high-speed blender and blend until smooth.

Yield: 2 servings

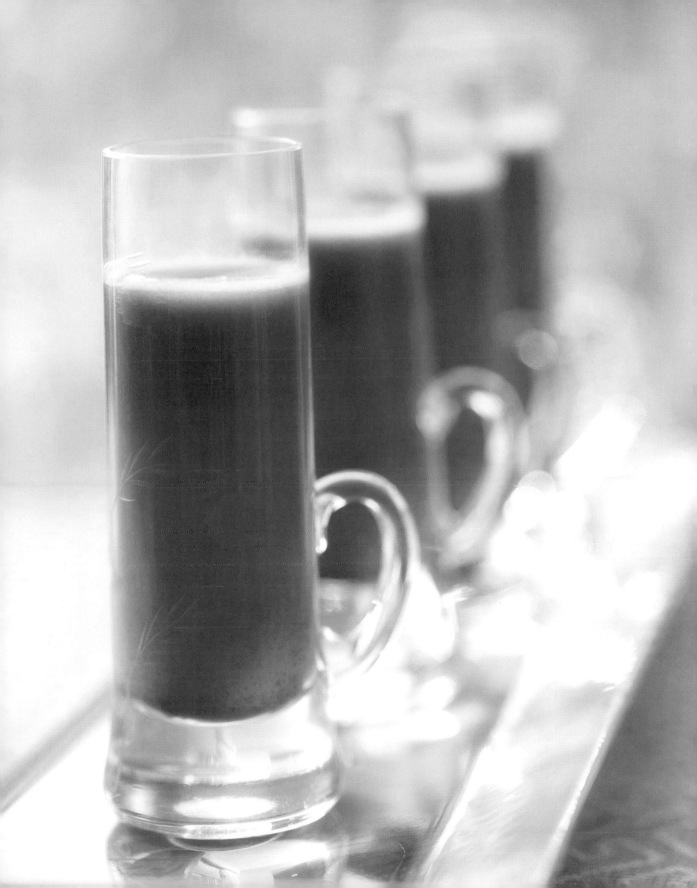

VINEGAR
Super Fermented Tonic

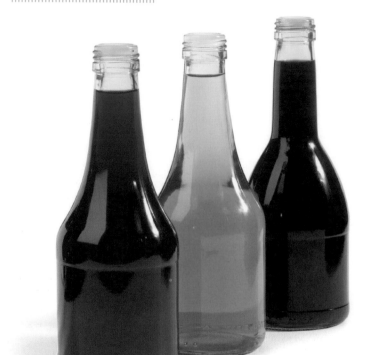

As a child of a large Italian family, my nearly every meal started—or ended—with a big salad tossed in a homemade vinaigrette. And along with a big salad, meals also included a large loaf (or two) of homemade Italian bread, which we used to soak up the dressing that remained on our salad plates long after the vegetables were gone. Back then, vinegar was a condiment that I suspected did little more than add a bit of flavor to our everyday meals. But I know now that the addition of vinegar to our often starch-based meals (think bread and

pasta) may have served a bigger purpose. Researchers are finding that vinegar may help regulate blood sugar levels, increase satiety, and perhaps even help us stay slim. It is a super tonic that is super simple to incorporate into our daily diets.

Vinegar Rich in Healthy Acetic Acid

Vinegar is a fermented food whose name comes from the French *vin aigre*, meaning "sour wine." It is made by fermenting any high-carbohydrate source—such as apples, grapes, or barley—with yeast to produce an alcohol. That alcohol is then further fermented by acetic acid bacteria (*Acetobacter*), which produces the product we know as vinegar. It may then undergo filtration and pasteurization, or in the case of raw apple cider vinegar, it remains raw, unfiltered, and unpasteurized, which is said to protect it from nutrient losses.

Vinegar May Help Control Blood Sugars at Mealtime

Vinegar has numerous potential health benefits that researchers have been exploring over the past decade or more. In animal studies, researchers have found that vinegar may help lower blood pressure, possibly because of acetic acid's ability to enhance the absorption of calcium and other minerals. And in cell studies, researchers have found that certain types of vinegar, such as rice and sugar cane, may inhibit the growth and proliferation of some cancer cells, including leukemia, and even shrink tumors, like those of the colon. But where researchers have seen some of the most profound benefits of vinegar is in the area of blood sugar control.

Vinegar has been described as antiglycemic, and researchers have found that it appears to delay gastric emptying rates (meaning food stays in the stomach longer), lower the glycemic index of meals (how quickly the meal will cause an increase in blood sugars), and decrease postmeal blood sugar and insulin levels—especially in meals that are rich in carbohydrates. And although researchers are not entirely clear on the mechanism through which vinegar exerts these beneficial effects, they speculate that the acetic acid somehow interferes with the enzymes involved in starch digestion.

In a study published in *Diabetes Care* in 2004, researchers looked at the effects of vinegar when consumed just prior to a carbohydrate-rich meal in healthy patients and those with diabetes or insulin resistance. They found that consuming vinegar—5 teaspoons (25 ml) of vinegar diluted with 5 teaspoons (25 ml) of water and 1 teaspoon of saccharin just a few minutes before mealtime, increased insulin sensitivity by 34 percent in those who were insulin resistant and by 19 percent in those with type 2 diabetes. They also found that all groups experienced reduced insulin levels following the meal, and that the insulin resistant and diabetic patients reduced blood sugar levels following the meal.

In a more recent study published in 2010, researchers at Arizona State University found that 10 grams (2 teaspoons) of vinegar helped reduce blood sugar levels after mealtime—particularly when the vinegar was consumed with the meal and the meal consisted of high complex carbohydrates (in this case, a bagel and orange juice).

Vinegar for Weight Control

Let me start by saying that vinegar is not a weight-loss miracle food. However, some compelling studies suggest that its addition to a meal helps promote satiety likely because of its ability to slow gastric emptying and lower the glycemic-index load of the meal—and if you are full, you are less likely to overeat. It may also help you consume fewer calories.

In a study published in 2005, researchers found that when vinegar was added to a high-carbohydrate breakfast (again, bagel and orange juice) it not only lowered the glycemic index of the meal, but it also influenced how subjects ate the remainder of the day. Subjects who included vinegar in the morning meal consumed, on average, 200 fewer calories each day than those who did not.

PUTTING IT INTO PRACTICE

Vinegar is a healthful food and appears to work best when consumed with meals—especially those that are carbohydrate-rich. And I recommend adding it to your meals in the form of a homemade dressing that can be used in salads and vegetables. Balsamic, apple cider, and rice vinegars are three of my favorites that can be used in nearly any homemade dressing or marinade. Rice vinegar combines nicely with sesame oil in Asian dishes, while balsamic and apple cider can be used to create dressings for salads and steamed or fresh vegetables. Simply combine vinegar and oil in a 1:3 ratio and add spices like freshly crushed garlic, basil, thyme, rosemary, sea salt, and pepper for added flavor.

The acetic acid in vinegar may also help promote weight loss. In a study published in 2009, researchers found that obese subjects who consumed acetic acid over a twelve-week period significantly decreased both their body weight and abdominal fat. And in another study published that year, researchers found that when rats were fed high-fat diets, those whose diet was supplemented with acetic acid gained 10 percent less body fat than those whose diet did not.

APPLE CIDER VINEGAR TONIC

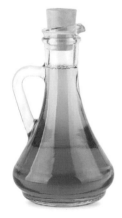

Because vinegar is so acidic, without proper dilution it may damage your skin, teeth, and esophagus. But when incorporated into salad dressings or added in small amounts to beverages—like this tart and tangy drink—it becomes a healthy and healing tonic.

2 to 3 apples
1½ cups (355 ml) filtered water
1 tablespoon (20 g) agave syrup
2 teaspoons raw apple cider vinegar
Ground cinnamon

Yield: 2 servings

Juice the apples. Blend the freshly pressed apple juice, water, agave syrup, and apple cider vinegar in a blender until combined. Alternatively, you can shake the ingredients together in a tightly lidded container or stir together in a large glass. Pour into one or two glasses (if sharing), sprinkle with cinnamon to taste, and serve.

RESOURCES

Food and Nutrition Information and Research

PubMed, U.S. National Library of Medicine, National Institutes of Health
www.ncbi.nlm.nih.gov/ pubmed

Contains more than 21 million citations for biomedical literature from MEDLINE, life science journals, and online books.

U.S. Department of Agriculture National Nutrient Database for Standard Reference
http://ndb.nal.usda.gov

Find nutrient information on nearly 8,000 foods with the ability to search by food item, group, or list to find nutrient information.

Local Food Resources

Co-op Directory Service
www.coopdirectory.org/ directory.htm

Edible Magazines
www.ediblecommunities.com

FarmersMarket.com
www.farmersmarket.com

Local Harvest
www.localharvest.org

Slow Food USA
www.slowfoodusa.org

Superfood Websites and Retailers

Amazing Grass
www.amazinggrass.com

Artisana
www.artisanafoods.com

Brad's Raw Food
www.bradsrawchips.com

Broccosprouts
www.broccosprouts.com

E3Live
www.e3live.com

Essential Living Foods
www.essentiallivingfoods. com

Genesis Today
www.genesistoday.com

GoHunza.com
www.gohunza.com

International Harvest, Inc.
www.internationalharvest. com

Kopali Organics
www.kopali.net

Lakewood Juices
www.lakewoodjuices.com

Live Superfoods
www.livesuperfoods.com

Living Intentions
www.shop.livingintentions. com

Manitoba Harvest
www.manitobaharvest.com

Navitas Naturals
www.navitasnaturals.com

Nutiva
www.nutiva.com

One Lucky Duck
www.oneluckyduck.com

Rhythm Superfoods
www.rhythmsuperfoods.com

Sacha Vida
www.sachavida.com

Sambazon
www.sambazon.com

Sibu
www.sibubeauty.com

Sproutman
www.sproutman.com

Sunfood Superfoods
www.sunfood.com

Wheatgrass Central
www.wheatgrasscentral.com

ACKNOWLEDGMENTS

With gratitude . . .

To my amazing husband, **Gary**, for your unconditional love and support throughout this project and always. You are my superman.

To my beautiful girl, **Maria**, for your endless love (and hugs), little Post-it notes of support, and laughter. You inspire me every day, little one.

To my parents, **Jim** and **Jo Ann**, and my sister, **Rebecca**, for a (mostly) slow food childhood. I'm grateful for days spent berry picking, gardening, composting, canning, and savoring thousands of made-from-scratch, sit-down meals (and family time) around the kitchen table.

To **Grandma Josephine** who would have been ninety-six at the time of this writing. I know you are watching over me in the kitchen and I miss you.

To **Cyndi Weis**, R.D., at Breathe Yoga—the space you have created in Breathe has inspired me both professionally and personally. I had my first green juice and açai breakfast bowl and took my first hot and sweaty yoga class at Breathe. I am grateful to be part of the community—thank you for all of your support.

To **Augusta Barstow** and **Denise Dube** for an amazing raw teacher weekend in Boston that inspired me to do more uncooking than cooking in my classes and kitchen. You girls are amazing!

To **Nil Zacharias**, **Preeta Sinha**, and **Daniel Lin** at One Green Planet for the opportunity to be part of such a wonderful online community helping to spread green living and veggie love. Thank you for your support.

To all of my beautiful friends for your friendship and support (and taste testing!). Especially **Gabrielle Javier-Cerulli**, M.A., author and expressive arts coach—you are no ordinary woman and a true master of the vision board. And **Trish Wager**, C.H.H.C., holistic health coach and partner in crime in all things food, yoga, meditation, and mala beads—you are a shining soul, my friend.

To **Christine Young** of the Handel Group, who helps me conquer the chicken and the brat each day so I have the space to accomplish my endeavors. Thank you for challenging me and for your continued support throughout this project.

To all of my **mentors** and **teachers** who have educated and inspired me over the years—and especially the students I have had the honor of working with. I wrote this book for all of you.

And finally, a huge thank you to my editors, **Jill Alexander**, **Cara Connors**, and **Renae Haines**—and everyone at Fair Winds Press—for giving this girl a dream job. I loved taking on this incredible topic and book, and I am grateful for the opportunity and for all of your guidance and support from start to finish.

ABOUT THE AUTHOR

Lauri Boone, R.D., is a food and nutrition expert, speaker, and writer. A registered dietitian specializing in plant-based nutrition, Lauri has worked in the nutrition and fitness fields since 1998. She has written for several publications and appeared in numerous media outlets including CNN, National Public Television, and *The Huffington Post*. Lauri is a regular contributor for *One Green Plant* and featured health expert on *ChickRx* and *Learn It Live*. She maintains a thriving private practice in upstate New York, where she lives with her husband, Gary, daughter, Maria, and rescue dog and cat, Lucky and Tom.

RECIPE INDEX

INDEX

INDEX